AIDS

AND THE
ARROWS OF PESTILENCE

AIDS

AND THE
ARROWS OF PESTILENCE

Charles F. Clark, M.D.

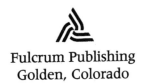

Fulcrum Publishing
Golden, Colorado

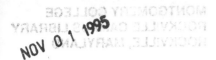

Permissions

Cover: *Tödlein* by Hans Leinberger, 1520. Used by permission of Kunsthistorisches Museum, Vienna.

Plate 1. Death cart figure by Nasario Lopez, late nineteenth century. Used by permission of Taylor Museum for Southwestern Studies of the Colorado Springs Fine Arts Center.

Plate 2. *The Plague in Rome*, from the "Legende Dores," Legend of St. Sebastian by Jules-Elie Delaunay, 1869. Used by permission of Erich Lessing/Art Resource, NY.

Plate 3. *Martyrdom of Saint Sebastian* by Giovanni del Biondo, 1350. Used by permission of Scala/Art Resource, NY.

Plate 4. *Saint Sebastian* by Sodoma, 1528. Used by permission of Scala/Art Resurce, NY.

Plate 5. *Saint Sebastian Protecting the Devoted from the Plague* by Benozzo Gozzoli, 1464. Used by permission of Scala/Art Resource, NY.

Plate 6. *Misericordia della Madonna* (Madonna of Mercy) by Benedetto Bonfigli, 1464. Used by permission of Scala/Art Resource, NY.

Plate 7. *Triumph of Death* by Pieter Brueghel (the Elder), 1556. Used by permission of Scala/Art Resource, NY.

Plate 8. Untitled by Brent Watkinson, 1992. Used by permission of Brent Watkinson, © 1994 Brent Watkinson.

Plate 9. *Der Tod als Kriegsknecht umfasst ein junges Mädchen* (Death, as a soldier [war-servant], embraces a young woman), by Niklaus Manuel Deutsch, 1517. Used by permission of Offentliche Kunstsammlung Basel, Kunstmuseum.

Plate 10. Untitled (illustration used on *Stern* magazine cover), by Nicholas Garland, 1988. Courtesy of *Stern*, Nicholas Garland and *The Spectator*.

Plate 11. AIDS Quilt (panels laid out on the Mall in Washington, D.C., International Display, October 1992), various dates; photograph by Mark Theissen. Used by permission of The NAMES Project Foundation and Mark Theissen.

Plate 12. AIDS Quilt (close-up of single panel), various dates; photograph by David Alosi and Ron Vak. Used by permission of David Alosi, Ron Vak and The NAMES Project Foundation.

Plate 13. Untitled (AIDS poster for ACT UP) by Keith Haring, 1989. Used by permission of The Estate of Keith Haring, © 1994 The Estate of Keith Haring.

Library of Congress Cataloging-in-Publication Data

Clark, Charles F.
    AIDS and the arrows of pestilence / Charles F. Clark.
        p.   cm.
    Includes bibliographical references (p.).
    ISBN 1-55591-146-3
    1. AIDS (Disease)—Social aspects.   2. AIDS (Disease)—History.
I. Title.
RA644.A25C53   1994
362.1'969792—dc20   94-11612
                                                                          CIP

Printed in the United States of America
Color signature printed in Korea

0 9 8 7 6 5 4 3 2 1

Fulcrum Publishing
350 Indiana Street, Suite 350
Golden, Colorado 80401-5093

For Carol, Joan, Brant and D'Aun

List of Plates

Cover: *Tödlein* by Hans Leinberger, 1520, Kunsthistorisches Museum, Vienna.

1. Death cart figure by Nasario Lopez, late nineteenth century, Colorado Springs Fine Arts Center.

2. *The Plague in Rome* by Jules-Elie Delaunay, 1869, Musee d'Orsay, Paris, France.

3. *Martyrdom of Saint Sebastian* by Giovanni del Biondo, 1350, Museo dell'Opera del Duomo, Florence, Italy.

4. *Saint Sebastian* by Sodoma, 1528, Galleria Palatina, Palazzo Pitti, Florence, Italy.

5. *Saint Sebastian Protecting the Devoted from the Plague* by Benozzo Gozzoli, 1464, Church of San Agostino, San Gimignano, Italy.

6. *Misericordia della Madonna* by Benedetto Bonfigli, 1464, Church of San Francesco del Prato, Perugia, Italy.

7. *Triumph of Death* by Pieter Brueghel (the Elder), 1556, Prado, Madrid, Spain.

8. Untitled by Brent Watkinson, 1992, private collection.

9. *Der Tod als Kriegsknecht umfasst ein junges Mädchen* by Niklaus Manuel Deutsch, 1517, Kunstmuseum, Basel, Switzerland.

10. Untitled (*Stern* magazine cover illustration), by Nicholas Garland, 1988.

11. AIDS Quilt (panels laid out on the Mall in Washington, D.C., International Display, October 1992), various dates; photograph by Mark Theissen, The NAMES Project Foundation.

12. AIDS Quilt (close-up of single panel), various dates; photograph by David Alosi and Ron Vak, The NAMES Project Foundation.

13. Untitled (AIDS poster for ACT UP) by Keith Haring, 1989, private collection.

Table of Contents

Acknowledgments

THE WORK OF PROFESSOR WILLIAM MCNEILL, as expressed in his book *Plagues and Peoples*, has shaped my thinking about our cultural experience with epidemic disease, including AIDS. Ten years in the making, this book elaborates some of his themes.

I was made aware of the seriousness of the AIDS epidemic by my associate, Presly Reed, before the epidemic had even been officially named. Robert Redfield taught me the biology of the virus. Chuck Kuhn helped me to examine the issues generated by the epidemic as we traveled through Europe on military duty. At the University of South Florida, Michael Knox supported my lectures, and his staff at the Center for HIV Education provided every assistance. Lois Nixon helped me to understand that we learn best through the medium of stories and that our history has been recorded by our artists. Mike Sample was my steadfast companion while tracking down obscure plague art in Europe and Asia. Author Jeff Long, a friend from my climbing days in the Himalayas, proposed that I write this book and patiently walked me through the entire process.

I am grateful for all the kind assistance I received from friends and colleagues and for the cheerful support of my family.

My editor David Nuss was thoughtful and diplomatic as he focused the book and enchanced the text. Photographs and permissions were all obtained through the inspired efforts of Heidi Herndon. My publisher Bob Baron and his staff enthusiastically embraced the manuscript and used their many talents to produce an aesthetically pleasing book.

In borrowing information from many different fields and weaving it into a manageable story, I have inevitably made some errors of fact and interpretation. Friends generously gave their time to identify and correct these and to criticize the manuscript. Any errors that remain are my own responsibility.

—*Charles F. Clark*
Tampa, April 3, 1994

Introduction

AIDS HAS BEEN IDENTIFIED in the public mind as a disease of specific marginalized groups in American society, initially gay men, then hemophiliacs and people who inject drugs and now black females and their children. How concerned should an individual be about the danger that the epidemic poses; how likely is it to have a significant effect on an individual's life?

Reputable scientists have questioned whether the AIDS virus, HIV, will ever establish itself among white, middle-class heterosexuals. Is there any real risk of the disease moving into the population of young heterosexuals with the implication that it would then disseminate into the general population? While there is the occasional story of the businessman who acquired the virus on the road and brought it home to his wife, the statistics, now in the hundreds of thousands, relentlessly demonstrate that the disease is concentrated among male homosexuals and other marginalized groups.[1] However, the possibility of spread within the heterosexual population is certainly present. Asia offers an example of what can happen. For years it was affected little by the epidemic. Then, in northern Thailand the rate of HIV infection in randomly tested male military draftees rose abruptly from 0.5 percent in 1989.[2] The rate reached 12 percent in 1991, primarily in the heterosexual population.[3] Could a similar phenomenon occur in America where 4 percent of male high school seniors have been treated for a venereal disease?[4]

Because individuals become ill, health is experienced as a personal issue. One by one we become sick and sometimes die. Tended by family and friends, our only connection to others who suffer the same disease is through brief residence in the same impersonal hospital. This remains true even when the disease is an epidemic that is slaying tens of thousands of our fellow citizens. During wartime, many people perish simultaneously in a mass public dying, and our national conscience acknowledges that we have a shared responsibility for ending the carnage and caring for the survivors. Epidemics invoke no such response. Indeed, epidemics provoke condemnation of those who are ill, and blame for having behaved in such a way as to invite the illness. During epidemics, the ill persons are cast in the role of public enemy and shunned, if not overtly condemned.

Infectious diseases, however, are phenomena of groups, not of individuals. Vulnerable persons acquire the infection because it exists in their group, and not because of any particular personal behavior. Control of an epidemic is achieved by changing the groups' vulnerability, perhaps with vaccines or environmental improvement such as clean water. It is not achieved by haranguing individuals to change particular personal behaviors. Infectious diseases exist in communities, and only by dealing with an epidemic as a concern of the entire community can it potentially be controlled. We have learned this lesson with cholera, smallpox, polio, measles, malaria and tuberculosis. We must learn it again for AIDS.

Historians have tended to overrate battles as determinants of history, and have underrated epidemics. Battles are dramatic and easy to document. Great masses of people have the same experience simultaneously, collectively and publicly. The winners enthusiastically record their heroic feats. Epidemic disease is experienced as messy, personal, individual defeat with some survivors, but no winners, and no heroes. But epidemics in the past, most less deadly than AIDS, have profoundly influenced the economics, arts, culture, politics and religion in western Europe and North America. AIDS promises to do the same.

Innumerable volumes recount the few modest battles between the Army Cavalry and Native Americans, yet it was largely disease, not bullets, that annihilated the Native Americans.[5] Imagine for a moment what America would be like if Native Americans had not died of imported infectious diseases.

They might far outnumber those of European origin, and we would have a racial mix of Native Americans to Caucasians much like the present racial mix of natives to Europeans in South Africa with its obvious political ramifications. And had the Native Americans not died of disease, there might have been no importation of black African slaves into North America. Perhaps there would have been no American Civil War. Epidemics have had a profound, largely unrecognized effect on our history. The current, unusually deadly, epidemic, AIDS, is producing such an effect on our current social well-being.

Too often we think of AIDS as being a consequence of individual behavior. The decision to engage in intercourse without a condom, the decision to share IV drug paraphernalia, the decision to have unprotected sex with a prostitute, all are personal behaviors that may lead to infection. But infection with the AIDS virus can occur with these personal behaviors only because the AIDS virus exists in epidemic proportions in the general population. If the AIDS virus were not present, intercourse without a condom would carry no special hazard to the practitioner, IV drugs would carry a risk only for hepatitis infection and unprotected sex with a prostitute would carry no greater risk than infection with herpes, syphilis or other, less deadly, venereal diseases. It is not individual personal behaviors that cause infection with HIV. It is that the AIDS virus inhabits our community of people in which these personal behaviors have long been common.

Those who took comfort in the belief that AIDS posed no threat to them because of their sexual restraint and avoidance of IV drugs must now face the threat of tuberculosis as a secondary epidemic generated by our community experience with AIDS.[6] After years of decline, tuberculosis is on the rise, and unlike AIDS, which can be avoided by not engaging in specific behaviors, tuberculosis is air borne. Inactive tuberculosis infections that the body can suppress indefinitely can become active infections because of the damage HIV does to the immune system. Inadequate drug treatment of many patients co-infected with HIV and TB has resulted in strains of tuberculosis (Multiple Drug Resistant or MDR-TB) resistant to most of our standard antibiotics. Infection with these TB strains carries a significant death rate even with excellent medical treatment. Breathing, an activity which is difficult to avoid, may now be hazardous to your health.

To understand the AIDS epidemic we must examine our historical and cultural experience with disease and plagues, and seek to explain AIDS as the most recent epidemic in a long series of epidemics that have afflicted humankind. AIDS is not a CIA experiment gone awry, nor a sudden strange biological mutation. The origin of AIDS is found in a long-known and well-studied family of animal viruses, the Lenti viruses. Its spread is a normal manifestation of the interaction of evolutionary biology and cultural development.

While we regard our response to the AIDS epidemic as "natural" and "spontaneous," it is highly directed by the past experience of our culture with epidemic disease. Many of our current beliefs about AIDS can be traced all the way back to the time of Moses and Homer. By examining some of the art, both literary and visual, that provides the record of human experience with epidemic disease, we can craft our own approach to the current crisis.

The AIDS epidemic will affect all of us collectively as a community, and it will affect many of us personally through the deaths of friends, family members and colleagues. We cannot escape its influence. It affects our health system, our immigration policy, our tax rates, our legislation, our impulse to charity, our prisons and our attitudes toward the homeless. It is an increasingly popular subject for our poets, authors and filmmakers. One cannot go a week without seeing a major story about AIDS on television or in the newspaper.

While we are impatiently waiting and hoping for the discovery of a cure, or for the development of a protective vaccine, we are not helpless in the face of this epidemic. The way we have organized ourselves as a culture at this particular time in history has made us vulnerable to invasion by the AIDS virus, but through understanding our cultural contributions to the epidemic, we have the ability to change them and so alter the course of the epidemic. It is the ultimate purpose of this book to provide some basis for that understanding and to make some suggestions about what we might do as a culture to mitigate the effect of the AIDS epidemic.

Notes

1. "Acquired Immunodeficiency Syndrome—Dade County, Florida, 1981–1990," *Morbidity and Mortality Weekly Report (MMWR)*, vol. 40, no. 29 (1991): 489–93.

2. T. D. Mastro, T. Nopkesorn and S. Sangkharomya, "HIV-1 Infection in Young Men in Northern Thailand," *AIDS*, vol. 7 (1993): 1233–39.

3. D. D. Celentano, K. E. Nelson and S. Suprasert, "Risk Factors for HIV Infection among Young Adult Men in Northern Thailand," *Journal of the American Medical Association*, vol. 270, no. 8 (1993): 955–60.

4. "Sexual Behavior Among High School Students—United States, 1990," *MMWR*, vol.40, no.51 (1992): 885–88.

5. Lesle Roberts, "Disease and Death in the New World," *Science*, vol. 246, no. 4935 (Dec. 8, 1989): 1245–47.

6. C. R. Horsburgh, Jr., and A. Pozniak, "The Epidemiology of Tuberculosis in the Era of HIV," *AIDS*, vol. 7, suppl. 1 (1993): S109–14.

AIDS

AND THE
ARROWS OF PESTILENCE

Chapter 1

In the Beginning ...
There Was Disease

WHETHER GUIDED BY THE HAND of God, the forces of survival or a roll of cosmic dice, humanity probably evolved from a common ancestor with the ape. The first humans who dropped out of the trees onto the placid and temperate African savanna several million years ago came to understand their mortality. Death, for them, most often came from infection or accident, not the infirmities of old age. Old age was so rarely achieved that the elderly were revered as wise and holy. They were believed to have been especially favored by God to have lived for so long.[1]

Early humans did not suffer from most of the diseases that are commonplace today. The illnesses that we experience could not have existed in early human society because there were too few people, too thinly spread, to support them. People were banded together in small groups of hunter-gatherers.[2] They ate nuts, berries and other edible plants, moving frequently in response to seasonally changing food supplies. In order for modern infectious diseases to exist in a population, a new susceptible person must enter the chain of infection every one to two weeks. To remain viable, the germs must constantly leap from one susceptible person to another. Within two weeks, the germs induce in the infected person a strong, lifelong immunity to that particular germ. The need for the rapid spread of modern diseases, such as measles, mumps, smallpox, flu or the common cold, requires a population density that cannot be supported by a hunting-and-gathering social organization.[3]

Today, the same phenomenon is regularly observed in scientific parties wintering in the Antarctic. After a one-month period during which everyone catches everyone else's cold, there are no more colds. Through the winter, there are no new infectious diseases. The wintering party has briefly reproduced the cultural circumstances of our distant ancestors. In the springtime, the relief personnel bring civilization in the form of supplies, equipment and new disease germs.

Although early humans never caught a cold, they were not disease free. Humans were susceptible to some of the diseases of the herd animals that they followed and hunted. Using the same water holes as the animals exposed humans to the same intestinal infections that the animals had. And humans were bitten by the same insects that bit animals. By these routes, early humans were exposed to infectious microorganisms, some of which were able to live in humans. If the germ found a reliable technique for transmission from one person to another, it could eventually evolve into a disease that lived exclusively in humans.

Chicken pox is an example of a virus that might have developed very early in human history.[4] It is able to flourish in small isolated social groupings such as those of early hunter-gatherers. It is easily spread by physical contact and will rapidly infect all susceptible individuals in a close, small community. However, although infection induces lifelong immunity, the immunity protects only against new infection; it does not protect against a recurrence of the old infection.

After the infection invokes an immune response, some of the chicken pox virus retreats to the nerve tissue of the infected person. There it is safe from the immune response that destroys the virus in the rest of the body. The virus hides, dormant, doing no harm and causing no symptoms. Then, when the infected person is perhaps forty or fifty years old, the virus breaks out of the nerve tissue and causes a highly infectious rash to develop on a small area of skin. This rash, called shingles, sheds huge amounts of virus and serves to infect the next generation. This elaborate, hibernation-like strategy is no longer necessary in modern, highly concentrated populations in which a virus can simply leap from one susceptible person to another.

The chicken pox virus evolved in order to survive in primitive human society. Indeed, every microorganism that causes an infectious disease of humans must have a specific and precise strategy for transmission and survival. Each must take advantage of some human physiological weakness or fundamental human behavior to ensure its reproductive success and transmission.

Malaria is another ancient disease. Its various forms—all transmitted by mosquitoes—infect reptiles and birds as well as mammals. Of the four types that infect humans, three cause only mild to moderate illness. Humans and the disease are well adapted to each other—we are a reliable host, and the disease does not make us very ill. The fourth type of human malaria, *Falciparum*, causes a severe illness in most people, frequently resulting in death. The people of some tribes in Africa developed partial protection against *Falciparum* malaria through the genetic selection of an abnormal sickle form of hemoglobin, the protein that carries oxygen inside the red blood cell. This genetic selection conveys resistance to infection by *Falciparum* malaria if one sickle gene is inherited; however, it also results in sickle cell anemia and death if two genes are inherited.

Many African tribes who have lived for many generations in an area infested with *Falciparum* malaria have adapted genetically and thus improved their survival.[5] But the price was high: a genetic mutation that is sometimes fatal. In an evolutionary sense, the cost is a trade-off. It enables the tribes to occupy areas of the earth that otherwise would be uninhabitable.

The chicken pox virus and *Falciparum* malaria provide examples of germs adapting in order to survive in humans, and humans adapting in order to control the intrusion of disease germs. The assault and the counterattack of disease microorganisms and their human hosts are always precise and specific.

Humans have some twenty years between generations. The Anopheles mosquito has a few months between generations. *Falciparum* malaria has just a few days. Since humans are at an obvious disadvantage in the race to evolve, genetic adaptations, such as the sickle hemoglobin, are not always viable defenses against disease organisms. We compensate for our biological slowness with cultural innovation. The struggle between the cultural innovations of humans and the genetic adaptations of disease microorganisms and insects is endless.[6]

The human struggle with *Falciparum* malaria and the Anopheles mosquito, its secondary host, continues. Modern humans have pitted cultural innovation, in the form of drugs and insecticides, against the biological adaptation of the microorganism and insect. We are not winning.[7] *Falciparum* malaria has developed resistance to most antimalarial drugs, and the Anopheles mosquito has developed resistance to most insecticides. The result of modern human intervention is that the disease and the insect have adapted genetically to create resistant varieties.

Humans, mosquitoes and malaria are in a competition, each changing to gain some advantage over the others. We have come to believe that nature, without the intervention of humans, would be in balance. In truth, nature is permanently out of balance. The pressure to select a mutatation that can expand the range and thus increase the population of any given species is tremendous. Each newly successful species changes its environment simply by existing. Selective evolutionary pressure on all living organisms causes them to repeatedly adapt to and then overrun their place and space. Other living organisms must then adapt genetically to the newly created conditions in order to survive. Those that cannot adapt rapidly enough become extinct. The ecological balance that is supported by environmentalists does not exist, and the ongoing process of elimination and creation of species is natural and normal.

Employing cultural adaptation, humans could compete more effectively for ecological niches than by relying solely on the much slower biological adaptive process.[8] But any advantage is inevitably temporary. Our very success creates new ecological niches for other disease germs. As we expand our population, these new niches guide the genetic selection of other disease microorganisms. The more successful humans have become in terms of population growth, the more we have increased our vulnerability to new infectious disease. We have created the conditions for new epidemics by changing the ways in which we live and love and work. AIDS is the most recent such epidemic that has found opportunities created by changes in our social structure.

If a disease germ can live in a newly found host and has some method of transmission from host to host, it will eventually develop a nonlethal form.[9] The most virulent strains, those that rapidly kill their host, stop their own transmission. When the host dies, they die too. The more benign strains allow their host to live, permitting their wide dissemination. The more benign strains of a disease germ become more common and more widely spread. The more virulent strains become less common and eventually disappear. Evolution thus favors the selection of the benign strains of a disease.

This same evolutionary process also favors the development of human resistance to a given disease. When the disease microorganism infects a host and the host lives, the host passes on to its offspring the characteristics that enabled it to survive the infection. When the microorganism infects a host and that host dies, that host has no offspring, and susceptibility to the infection is not passed on to the next generation. Instead, it is eliminated from the host species. This selects for disease resistance in the host species. This phenomenon selected sickle hemoglobin in Africans in response to the pressure of *Falciparum* malaria infection.

This evolutionary pressure on the germ to produce less severe illness, and this evolutionary pressure on the host for greater disease resistance, causes diseases to constantly change in their appearance. This makes it difficult to identify the germs that caused ancient epidemics. The appearance of a disease will change as the germ ages. Ultimately, the disease germ and host may so adapt to each other that the presence of the microorganism does not cause any illness unless the natural resistance of the host is greatly reduced for some reason. In general, the longer a disease has been around, the milder it is. Diseases that kill a high percentage of infected persons are generally so new that humans have not had a chance to adapt biologically. AIDS is such a new disease.

When primitive humans journeyed north out of the cradle of Africa, they came to a colder, dryer climate. Fewer insects and germs could survive the cold, so there was less infectious disease. But the cold of winter was also harsh. To survive in a cold climate, humans had to conserve heat. One response was genetically adaptive—over many millenia and an ice age, humans became hairier. The pressures of a new environment also forced humans to adapt culturally. They learned to kill animals and use the skins as warm clothing. They developed the spear. They first learned to conserve a natural fire and to carry it from place to place, then, eventually, learned how to spark and build a fire.

Domestication of animals and the development of agriculture allowed changes in social organizaton, making it possible for more people to live in smaller areas. Population density, in turn, supported diversification of occupations and the development of civilization. It also increased the vulnerability of the more densely organized human population to new infectious disease. This human cultural adaptability greatly expanded the area of the earth that people could occupy. However, each time we moved into a new area, we were exposed to new disease germs. Our vulnerability to infectious disease increasingly became determined by the way we organized and spread our culture. As civilization evolved, so did human disease.

Many of the animals domesticated by humans were herd animals that are subject to epidemics. Humans lived in close daily contact with animals and were constantly exposed to their diseases.[10] This intense level of exposure was much greater than humans had experienced as hunters. Man's "best friend," the dog, has given him at least sixty-five diseases. Altogether, domesticated animals and rats and mice have given humans at least 250 diseases.[11] Some disease germs that have crossed over into humans have probably been so altered by selective evolutionary pressure that their origins are no longer recognizable. Thus, any estimate of human diseases acquired from domesticated animals is almost certainly too low.[12]

The development of agriculture also created another critical cultural problem for humans.[13] By staying in one place, humans created problems of contaminated water and a buildup of human waste, which in turn supported diseases like cholera, typhoid fever and schistosomiasis.

After each cultural advance, the human population rose, then fell with each new disease, then rose again as humans and the disease microorganisms adapted to each other.[14] Humans had clearly escaped from the constraints imposed by biology, altering their environment and culture to meet their needs.

As villages grew in number and in size, and specialized occupations developed, area trade increased and some villages, favored by location or by unusually competent leadership, grew faster and larger than the others. They came to dominate their geographical areas and became the first cities. Approximately six thousand years ago the population of these cities, and of the surrounding areas, finally provided a pool of humans that was large enough to support modern diseases.[15] There were now enough humans in constant contact with one another that modern disease germs, such as smallpox, measles, mumps, flu and the common cold, would always have susceptible humans available for infection.

Cultural advances did not occur in all parts of the world simultaneously. Some populations advanced rapidly, others slowly and others not at all. The world was so large, and travel so difficult, that some societies grew to be powerful and populous states and yet had no contact with other great states. Population densities varied widely. Some societies offered greater opportunities for the introduction and survival of infectious diseases than did others. Diverse disease microorganisms crossed over into humans in different places and at different times. The infected humans and the invading microorganisms responded to the selective evolutionary pressure and adapted to each other. The selection for natural disease resistance occurred only in the humans who lived in the area of a particular disease. All the other humans in the world remained naïve, and therefore vulnerable to deadly infection.

Travel by humans from one city to another thus carried the threat of epidemic disease.[16] Disease microorganisms began to leak through the geographical barriers. Four great centers of human population had developed by the time of the Roman Empire: Sub-Saharan Africa, where humans had originated; northern India; northern China and the Mediterranean Basin. Each population center had developed its own unique pool of infectious diseases.[17] The consequences of mixing those disease pools would dominate human history for a thousand years.

Caesar Augustus, Emperor of Rome, had begun the Pax Romana, the Roman Peace, by force of arms. Under it, trade and commerce flourished from Britain in the West to India and China in the East and to Ethiopia in the South. In the center was Rome, trading capital of the world. The trade in goods inevitably carried with it a trade in ideas, religions and diseases. The Pax Romana fostered the trade that made Rome great. It then destroyed Rome with the inadvertent introduction of deadly epidemic diseases.

The first pestilential disaster to strike the Roman Empire, the "Plague of Antonius" in A.D. 165, appears to have been smallpox.[18] The description given by contemporary chroniclers of the manifestations of this disease permits us to be reasonably confident of the diagnosis. This is not the smallpox we have known in the twentieth century. This was smallpox infecting a population that was naïve both biologically and culturally. The disease had probably come from India. Hindu religious writing and visual art suggest that it had long been a disease of that subcontinent. Overland trade had brought it to the Middle East, and a Roman army acquired it there while subduing the Parthian revolt in what is now Iran. When the Roman General, Lucius Verus, led his triumphant army back from Babylon to Rome, he brought with him the "Great Pest"— smallpox. The "Plague of Antonius" killed some 30 percent of the Roman population.

In A.D. 251, during the reign of Aurelius, another great plague struck Rome.[19] This is thought to have been measles— not the measles of the twentieth century, a febrile two-week illness of childhood, but a new disease, hitting a naïve population. Again, the population was devastated—10 to 20 percent died.

Smallpox and measles continued to ravage the population of the Roman Empire for 150 years, hitting hardest in the western provinces, and causing the population to decline sharply. In A.D. 330, the consequences of this series of epidemics prompted the Emperor Constantine to move the capital of the Roman Empire from Rome to the previously Greek city of Byzantium (which became Constantinople and is now Istanbul) in the more populous East.

With the aggregate population of the Roman Empire in both the East and West large enough to maintain both smallpox and measles, resistance to the diseases by natural selection began to slowly develop while the many deaths kept the population well below what the land could support under Roman techniques of farming, trade and industry. The western provinces remained so sparsely populated they were difficult to defend from Germanic tribes. The city of Rome was sacked by the Goths in A.D. 410 and plundered by the Vandals in A.D. 455. The last Roman ruler of the western provinces, Romulus, was deposed by the German chief Odoacer in A.D. 476. With the assimilation of these Germanic conquerors into Roman civilization, as well as the increasing resistance of the populace to disease, the population of the western provinces began to increase.

Just as Emperor Justinian made plans to return the capital of the Roman Empire to Rome, however, an infectious disease once again changed the course of history.[20] In A.D. 542, what appears from the description of the contemporary historian Procopius to have been *Pasteureila pestis*, bubonic plague, devastated the empire, both east and west. [21] That epidemic destroyed the resurgent power of Rome.[22] Justinian was not able to move the capital under such dire conditions, and the Roman Empire in the West disintegrated.

With the population base and trading system that had enabled Rome to dominate southern Europe, the Middle East and North Africa destroyed, Europe entered the Dark Ages. Ravaged by disease and pestilence, the empire fractured into multiple small economic and language units dominated by subsistence agriculture and regressive political processes. Generations passed, and the population adapted through natural selection to the diseases brought to Europe by Roman civilization. Life, however, remained dirty, harsh and generally brief.

In A.D. 610 as Europe adjusted to the new diseases and slept in the embrace of the Roman Catholic Church, the desert gave birth to another religion, Islam. The pagan tribesmen of the Arabian desert, converted by a merchant to a belief in the God of the Jews, and armed with a promise of direct admission to heaven for those who died in His service, swept the known world before them. They conquered North Africa, crossed the Straits of Gibraltar and marched north through Spain until halted by the army of Charles Martel at the Battle of Tours, France, in A.D. 732. From the desert of the Arabian Peninsula, the armies of the Muslim faithful also went east, taking Persia, Afghanistan and northern India. They struck northeast, conquering the steppes of Asia, Mongolia and northern China. To the north and west, the armies of the faithful eventually conquered the Balkans and even besieged Vienna. The siege was lifted when the deadly infectious disease, typhus, destroyed the army of Islam and halted its advance into Europe.

The Muslims thus conquered nations and acquired land, knowledge and ideas—and diseases. Their empire exceeded that of Rome's in size, although they never controlled their territory as effectively. They became the successors to the intellectual traditions of the Greeks and Romans. Science and the arts flourished in their cities.

Epidemic disease struck repeatedly in the Muslim lands. The farflung empire and its extensive trade assured the continued integration of the African, Indian, Chinese and Mediterranean disease pools, but while epidemics were frequent in the Islamic lands, the Muslim peoples never experienced anything as devastating as the plagues that destroyed the Roman Empire, or the Black Death which was to overwhelm Europe. This suggests that a broad and ill-defined cultural effect of the teachings of Mohammed somehow inhibited epidemic disease. The Islamic belief that God determines all events led to a passive response to epidemics, but such beliefs also emphasized that one must neither enter nor leave an area in which plague raged.[23] This had the beneficial effect of limiting the spread of an epidemic, because it was sacreligious to flee in an effort to save one's life.[24] Such beliefs did not prevent epidemic disease from ravaging local areas, but they did prevent epidemics from suddenly sweeping the entire Islamic Empire.

In 1071, Seljak Turks captured Jerusalem and began to harass Christian pilgrims. They threatened the existence of the shrunken Eastern or Byzantine Roman Empire, with its capital at Constantinople. The Byzantine Roman emperor, Commenus, asked for assistance in fighting the Seljek Turks from the Roman Pope, Urban II, temporal ruler of Rome and the Papal States, This help took the form of the Crusades, which consisted of eight military and political expeditions from Europe to the Eastern Mediterranean between 1096 and 1270. The First Crusade recaptured Jerusalem and the coast to the north. Subsequent Crusades had more to do with politics in Europe than with protecting the Christians in Jerusalem and ultimately had their greatest effect on Europe through the discovery of the goods, the commerce and the ideas of a larger world. The sleep of Europe, the Dark Ages, was over.

Marco Polo's famous journey to China in 1271 to visit the Kublai Khan was along a route that had been abandoned for a thousand years, the Roman Silk Road. His remarkable adventure presaged the reestablishment of trade and commerce between the East and the West. Ideas and disease would shortly follow. The most devastating epidemic in the history of the West would come from the East on the trading ships of the Italian city-states.

"The Pest," or as we know it, the Black Death, entered recorded history at the Genoese trading town of Caffa in 1346. Built on the Crimean Peninsula, which juts southward into the Black Sea, Caffa was an Italian commercial opening to the goods of the central Asian steppe. A Mongol army besieging that trading town was suddenly struck by a strange and lethal pestilence. The army abruptly withdrew, but not before the town was infected. Many in the town fled the pestilential catastrophe, unwittingly carrying "the Pest" to the other ports on the Black Sea, and then into the Mediterranean. 1348 was a terrifying year for the people of Europe.[25] Strange and agonizing death struck many thousands of people. There was no obvious explanation for who would become ill, and, for those who would die.

We know now that the offending germ was *Pasteureila pestis*, which was carried by fleas that infested rats and humans.[26] When an infected rat or human died and the body began to cool, the fleas would seek a new host. Thus the disease spread from one person to another and from one town to another.

By the fourteenth century, the population in Europe had expanded to the limits of the available technology.[27] Farmers had been forced to cultivate marginal land because the food-producing capacity of the good land had been exceeded. The cities had outgrown the limits of food and water distribution and sewage disposal. Housing was primitive and inadequate. The standard of living and the nutritional status were falling for all except the landed gentry and churchmen. Living conditions in the fourteenth century were overcrowded and filthy, and fleas abounded on both animals and humans. The social structure and cultural organization of Europe made it extremely vulnerable to a new disease spread by such conditions.

In 1348, *Pasteureila pestis* killed a fourth of the population of Europe. For the next three hundred years, "the Pest" repeatedly swept through Europe on an irregular schedule, averaging about every ten years. It reduced and then held the population down until the seventeenth century, when social changes decreased crowding, filth, and fleas. Europe's vulnerability to "the Pest" diminished, then ceased. The last attack of "the Pest" occurred in Marseilles, France, in 1720.[28] It has never recurred in Europe despite the presence of fleas, rats and the *Pasteureila* germ. Improved living standards prevent a recurrence.

The next great mixing of disease pools began with the discovery of the New World by Christopher Columbus in 1492.[29] Conquest and subsequent coloniziation by Europeans exposed the native population to the pooled diseases of Africa, Europe and Asia. The result was death at a truly horrific rate for Native Americans.[30]

The New World also had its own disease pool. The most devastating Native American disease that was transmitted to the peoples of the Old World was syphilis.[31] That venereal disease came to Spain in 1493 with the returning crew from the first voyage of Christopher Columbus to the West Indies.[32] Syphilis came to be known in Europe as the Great Pox. This distinguished it from that other killer pox, smallpox. Syphilis was taken to Italy from Spain in 1496 in the army of Ferdinand and Isabella, sent to defend Naples from the mercenary army of Phillip V, King of France. Phillip conquered the city of Naples, and his soldiers then carried the disease all over Europe as they returned to their homes after the campaign. Within ten years, the disease had reached India and China.

When the Spanish Conquistador Hernando Cortez attacked the Aztec Empire in 1519 with some six hundred men armed with primitive guns, a civilization of many millions opposed him. Remarkably, however, Cortez was victorious, for in addition to a suicidal courage, he had also brought smallpox.[33] In a single year smallpox killed 20 to 30 percent of the Aztec people. That left more than enough Aztecs to have annihilated Cortez and his band many times over. But the devastating epidemic killed most of the Aztec leadership and demoralized the people.

The Inca Empire fell under similar circumstances to another adventurer, Francisco Pizarro. With the further introduction of measles, typhus, mumps and yellow fever, the native populations of Mexico, Central America and South America almost vanished. Their languages, religions and cultures almost disappeared under the onslaught of Europeans and new epidemic diseases.

North of the Rio Grande, the absence of large native empires restricted the spread of the new epidemic diseases.[34] A slower annihilation of the native population occurred as each individual Indian tribe came into close contact with the Europeans. Overall, the Native Americans were subdued not by military might, but by the pooled diseases of Europe, Africa and Asia. Guns and the perfidy of the Europeans reduced the native North and South American populations only slightly. The near disappearance of the native people was almost entirely due to disease.[35]

Similar events marked the colonization of Africa, only this time it was the colonizers who suffered. When Africa was colonized by the Europeans, the native people did not die from newly introduced diseases. Africans already belonged to the same disease pool as the colonizing Europeans because trade with Africa had begun during the Roman Empire. Yet while the black Africans had adapted to all of the infectious diseases that existed in Europe, there were some infectious diseases native to Africa that had never become established in Europe because their insect vectors could not survive the European winters. The Europeans were biologically and culturally naïve to diseases such as sleeping sickness and yellow fever, and they died from them in large numbers.

North and South America and Africa were colonized at about the same time by white Europeans. Africa continues to this day to have blacks as the dominant population. In the Americas, the Indians almost died out, to be replaced by Europeans and Africans. Most history books do not mention disease in their accounts of the conquest of the Americas. There is a simple explanation. Those who conquer territory believe that they do so through bravery and skill, and they are the ones who write the history books. Those who lose because of disease and other causes are usually dead; they leave no record of why they lost.

Notes

1. W. S. Arnett, "Only the Bad Died Young in the Ancient Middle East," *International Journal of Aging and Human Development*, vol. 21, no. 2 (1985): 155–60.

2. The early development of humans and their interaction with disease is explained in Chapter 1 in *Plagues and Peoples*, William H. McNeil. (New York: Penguin Books, 1976). Anyone with a serious interest in understanding the interaction of infectious disease and human culture should read this book.

3. F. L. Black, "Measles Endemicity in Insular Populations: Critical Community Size and Its Evolutionary Implications," *Journal of Theoretical Biology*, vol. 11, no. 2 (July 1966): 207–11.

4. McNeil, *Plagues and Peoples*, 53.

5. Charlotte J. Avers, *Genetics* (New York: D. Van Nostrand Co, 1980), 600–601.

6. MacFarlane Burnet and David O. White, "Antibiotics," *Natural History of Infectious Diseases*. 4th ed. (New York: Cambridge University Press, 1972): 173–85.

7. J. E. Bennett, R. G. Douglas and G. L. Mandell, eds., *Principles and Practice of Infectious Diseases*, 2nd ed. (New York: John Wiley and Sons, 1985), 1514–15.

8. T. R. Southwood, "The Natural Environment and Disease: An Evolutionary Perspective," *British Medical Journal—Clinical Research*, vol. 294, no. 6579 (April 25, 1987): 1086–89.

9. MacFarlane Burnet and David O. White, "Evolution and Survival of Host and Parasite," *Natural History of Infectious Diseases*. 4th ed. (New York: Cambridge University Press, 1972), 137–54.

10. McNeil, *Plagues and Peoples*, 54–56.

11. Thomas G. Hull, ed., "The Role of Different Animals and Birds in Diseases Transmitted to Man," *Diseases Transmitted from Animals to Man*, 5th ed. (Springfield, Illinois: Charles C. Thomas, Publishers, 1963), 876–924.

12. D. L. Elliot, L. Goldberg, J. B. Miller and S. W. Tolle: "Pet-Associated Illness," *New England Journal of Medicine*, vol. 313, no. 16 (Oct. 17, 1985): 985–95.

13. McNeil, *Plagues and Peoples*, 45–47.

14. Bollet, Alfred J. "The Rise and Fall of Disease," *American Journal of Medicine*, vol. 70, no. 1 (January 1981): 12–16.

15. McNeil, *Plagues and Peoples*, 64.

16. The mixing of the disease pools and the effect of new diseases on the Roman Empire is explained in "Confluence of the Civilized Disease Pools of Eurasia: 500 B.C. to A.D. 1200," McNeil, *Plagues and Peoples*, 78–141.

17. McNeil, *Plagues and Peoples*, 108–12.

18. Donald R. Hopkins, "The Most Terrible of All the Ministers of Death," *Princes and Peasants, Smallpox in History* (Chicago: University of Chicago Press, 1983), 22.

19. McNeil, *Plagues and Peoples*, 113.

20. Ibid., 119.

21. Raymond Crawfurd, *Plague and Pestilence in Literature and Art* (Oxford: Clarendon Press, 1914), 77, 78.

22. John L. Dusseau, "The Plague: On the Evil and on the Good, on the Just and on the Unjust," *Perspectives in Biology and Medicine*, vol. 26, no. 1 (Autumn 1982): 46–50.

23. N. Alloush and W. B. Ober, "The Plague at Granada: 1348–1349: Ibn Al-Khatib and Ideas of Contagion," *Bulletin of the New York Academy of Medicine*, vol. 58, no. 4 (May 1982): 418–24.

24. Michael W. Dols, *The Black Death in the Middle East* (Princeton, New Jersey: Princeton University Press, 1977), 109–21.

25. Colin McEvedy, "The Bubonic Plague," *Scientific American*, vol. 258, no. 2 (February 1985): 118–23.

26. S. R. Ell, "Some Evidence for Interhuman Transmission of Medieval Plague," *Reviews of Infectious Diseases*, vol. 1, no. 3 (May–June, 1979): 563–66.

27. The effect of this new epidemic of *Pastureila pestis* upon the culture of Europe is told in "Impact of the Mongol Empire on Shifting Disease Balances," McNeil, *Plagues and Peoples*, 141–84.

28. McEvedy, "The Bubonic Plague," in *Scientific American*, 188–223.

29. The effect of the introduction of Old World diseases on the native American populations is described in "Conquistador y Pestilencia," Alfred W. Crosby, Jr., *The Columbian Exchange, Biological and Cultural Consequences of 1492* (Westport, Connecticut: Greenwood Press, 1972), 35–64.
    The mixing of the Old World and New World disease pools is described in "Transoceanic Exchanges, 1500–1700," McNeil, *Plagues and Peoples*, 185–216.

30. Lesle Roberts, "Disease and Death in the New World," *Science*, vol. 246, no. 4935 (December 8, 1989): 1245–47.

31. The effect of syphilis, a New World disease, on the population of Europe is described in "The Early History of Syphilis: A Reappraisal," Crosby, *The Columbian Exchange*, 122–64.

32. William B. Ober, "To Cast a Pox, the Iconography of Syphilis," *American Journal of Dermatopathology*, vol. 11, no. 1 (Feb. 1989): 74–86.

33. Crosby, "Conquistador y Pestilencia," *The Columbian Exchange*, 35–64.

34. Max Landsberger, "Communicable Diseases Across the Oceans," *New York State Journal of Medicine*, vol. 75, no. 9 (August 1975): 1568–75.

35. Henry F. Dobyns, *Their Number Became Thinned* (Knoxville: University of Tennessee Press, 1983).
S. F. Cook, "The Significance of Disease in the Extinction of the New England Indians," *Human Biology*, vol. 45, no. 3 (Sept. 1973): 485–508.

Chapter 2

The Arrows of Pestilence:
A Brief Iconology of Epidemic Disease

OUR UNDERSTANDING OF THE AIDS EPIDEMIC, with its intimate association with sex and death, is strongly influenced by our religious and artistic heritage. Many of our ideas about AIDS, and about those who suffer from AIDS, are derived directly from the past experience of our culture with deadly epidemic diseases. Today, our knowledge of our own artistic and cultural traditions regarding epidemic disease is somewhat limited because we have not experienced any devastating epidemics for several generations, and so we have not had any reason to develop that knowledge. We are generally not aware that our attitudes toward those with AIDS have been strongly influenced by the beliefs and legends of our ancestors.

Sex, love and death are entwined with one another through the symbol of the arrow in western European art. The arrow represents both love and pestilential disease. Our English word "toxin," meaning poison, is derived from the Greek word, "toxikon" (originally toxikon pharmakon, literally "bow poison," or "arrow").

In the *Iliad*, Homer recounts that Paris, son of Priam, the king of Troy, was visiting Sparta when he fell in love with Helen, the wife of his host, King Menelaus. She reciprocated, and Paris carried her home to Troy. Menelaus and his allies crossed the Aegean Sea to fight, and, if necessary, to die to reclaim this beautiful woman. History knows this quarrel between Helen's lovers and their respective allies as the Trojan War, and historians date the hostilities to about 1200 B.C.

The Greek attack, however, was stymied by the thick walls that surrounded the city of Troy. With nothing to do but wait for the defenders of Troy to sally forth for infrequent, brief and indecisive skirmishes, the great warrior leader of the Greeks, Agamemnon, grew bored and sexually frustrated. He kidnapped Chryseis, the daughter of the priest at the Shrine of Apollo, and despite the pleas of her father and his own companions-in-arms, refused to free her.

This abuse of the priest's daughter angered Apollo. To teach the Greeks a lesson, Apollo sent a terrible shower of arrows among them, manifested as a deadly sickness—a plague—that first killed the Greeks' dogs, then their horses and, finally, the warriors themselves. After Agamemnon returned the girl to her father, the pestilence ceased. Apparently because of this famous story, arrows came to symbolize the transmission of deadly disease epidemics.

Cupid, the god of love equipped with a bow and arrow, appears in the Greek play *Medea*. The playwright, Euripides, tells how Jason escaped with the Golden Fleece through the help of his lover Medea who had borne his two sons. When his love wandered to another woman, Medea in her anguish slew both of their children. Medea claimed her experience of love as a terrible sickness that she had acquired through Cupid's arrows. Our expression "lovesick" derives from the representation of love as a disease spread by arrows which are shot by Cupid.

The idea that disease, particularly epidemic disease, was sent from heaven also occurred to the followers of monotheism in the desert of the Middle East. The idea that the God of the Hebrews, Christians and Muslims inflicts disease on humans for punishment or instruction is firmly rooted in the *Pentateuch* (the first five books of the Old Testament). The best-known examples are the ten plagues visited upon the Egyptians during the time of Moses. These plagues, sent by God to instruct and punish the Egyptians, convinced the pharaoh to allow Moses and his people to depart from Egypt. The God of the Hebrews also sent disease onto his chosen people, collectively and individually, as instruction and punishment. Indeed, pestilence has been invoked in western culture for centuries as an example of God's will at work. Today, when a religious leader of one of three major religions—Judaism, Christianity and Islam—proclaims that AIDS is a plague sent by God, he or she gives voice to a recurring theme in western cultural heritage.

Hebrews believed that God's affliction of a person with disease demonstrated God's interest in that person. In a sense, God was *in* the sick person. Hebrews also felt a moral obligation to visit and to care for the sick, because God was interested in sick people. This duty was to be undertaken even at the risk of personal safety.[1] Judging a person and inflicting illness upon her or him were God's prerogatives. Visiting and caring for the sick were human duties. This included the care of sick gentiles and the care of those whose illness was attributed to sinful behavior.

The early followers of Jesus believed that he had extended the obligation of service, and made suffering while caring for or saving another person a route to special grace. It was not the suffering itself that brought grace, but rather the suffering while serving and saving other people.[2]

When smallpox came to Rome in A.D. 165 as the Plague of Antonius, tens of thousands of people were stricken, and many were abandoned by family, friends and physicians. With smallpox, as with measles and most other infectious diseases, mortality is considerably reduced if the patients receive supportive care and kind treatment. The early Christians fulfilled their belief in good works and personal sacrifice by visiting and caring for those stricken with deadly disease.[3] Many Romans were nursed back to health by Christians during the smallpox and measles epidemics.[4] This humanitarian aid was given freely and without expectation of earthly reward. Roman citizens converted to Christianity not to be martyred by being eaten by lions, but because the Christians were good, kind people who not only looked after one another, but even looked after strangers during times of epidemics.

Today, many of our hospitals belong to religious organizations. Every major city has a Jewish hospital and several belonging to Christian sects. These hospitals are the logical outcome of the religious beliefs and obligations of Jews and Christians, which stress care of the ill regardless of their beliefs or practices.

If one invokes the Judaic/Christian/Muslim tradition of God's punishment to explain the HIV epidemic, then perhaps, one should also invoke the tradition that true believers are to care for the sick and the dying. Jewish tradition makes clear the correct behavior toward the sick. Christians have the tradition of serving the sick, even at great personal risk, to emulate the willingness of Christ to suffer and die while serving and saving humankind. Muslims also have a special obligation to sick persons. The HIV epidemic has provided a marvelous opportunity to demonstrate moral courage, compassion and the Judaic/Christian/Muslim religious faith.

In the iconography of epidemic disease in western European art, the dominant plague figure is Saint Sebastian.[5] Most major museums possess one or more of his images. He is typically portrayed as a nearly nude young man with arrows piercing his body. Sometimes, as in Michaelangelo's representation in the Sistine Chapel, he is simply holding a bundle of arrows. The invocation of Saint Sebastian in time of disease is not merely a curiosity of history. His images may be purchased today in many Roman Catholic areas as talismans to ward off disease. Sebastian was also a figure in the Santos art of northern New Mexico in the early years of this century. Isolation of that culture is the apparent explanation for his conversion into a female skeletal figure shooting arrows from a "death cart"—a half-size wagon filled with stones that was pulled by a penitent of the Brotherhood of Jesus Christ during the Easter celebrations (see Plate One).[6]

Although Sebastian is known to have existed historically, the factual details of his life and death are uncertain. Whether fact or myth, Sebastian's story had great impact on western European ideas about epidemic disease. Born to Christian parents in third century Gaul, now France, Sebastian was raised in Milan. As a young adult, he moved to Rome and became a captain in the Praetorian Guard of the Emperor Diocletian. Several Christian friends were caught in one of the many persecutions, and Sebastian urged them not to recant their faith despite the threat of torture and death. This exposed his own Christian beliefs, and the emperor ordered him to be killed by archers. Wounded by arrows and left for dead, Sebastian was discovered by Christian friends and nursed back to health. This miraculous recovery from arrow wounds became the basis for the belief in his power against the plague as the plague was symbolically represented in Greek mythology by arrows.[7]

While Sebastian was convalescing at a home in Rome, he saw Diocletian approaching on the street. Sebastian berated the emperor for his treatment of the Christians. Diocletian was momentarily stunned because he had thought Sebastian was dead but soon regained his composure and ordered Sebastian beaten to death on the spot. Sebastian's body was cast into the *cloaca maxima,* the main sewer of Rome.

Christian companions learned in dreams where the body could be found. They recovered it and buried it south of Rome on the Appian Way in the catacomb that now bears Sebastian's name. We know from the writings of Saint Ambrose, Bishop of Milan in the fourth century, that Sebastian's tomb was already a site of pilgrimage at that time although it is not known if he was already connected symbolically with epidemic disease.[8]

The writings of John the Deacon, an eighth-century English monk, positively connected Saint Sebastian to epidemic disease.[9] Through his writings, we know that the seventh-century mosaic of Sebastian in the Church of Saint Peter in Chains in Rome was created to stop an epidemic. John the Deacon lived at the monastery of Monte Cassino and wrote a history of the Lombards, a Germanic tribe that had invaded and then settled in the Italian peninsula. In that history, he recounted the story of an epidemic that swept Rome in A.D. 683. That the epidemic was sent by God seemed obvious to everyone, for, according to the account, an angel of the Lord was seen going down the street and directing the "marking" by a "pest fiend" of the house doors of those who would die of the plague. This account is reflected in the dramatic painting by Jules-Elie Delaunay, who recorded the event on canvas in 1869(see Plate Two).

John the Deacon further related that during this epidemic there was a revelation about what was needed to halt the disease. The relics (bones) of Saint Sebastian were to be brought in a great procession from his tomb on the Appian Way to the Church of Saint Peter in Chains. They were to be placed in an altar dedicated to his memory. Some of his relics were promptly moved in the specified manner, and a new chapel decorated with a mosaic in his likeness was built. According to John the Deacon, the pestilence then ceased. Saint Sebastian came to symbolize hope and courage during times of epidemic disease.

The importance of such processions to convince God to halt punishment by pestilence was derived from the experience of Pope Gregory the Great in the latter part of the sixth century. The Roman Empire had been devastated by a terrible pestilence that began during the reign of the Emperor Justinian.[10] In A.D. 593, Pope Gregory led an enormous procession of citizens through the streets of Rome to demonstrate and pray for an end to the epidemic. During that procession, Pope Gregory reported seeing a vision of the Archangel Michael above the tomb of Hadrian on the banks of the River Tiber. Michael was sheathing his flaming sword, signifying to Gregory that God had ended the plague.

Today, there is bronze statue on the roof of the Tomb of Hadrian depicting the Archangel Michael sheathing his sword. Since the tenth century, the building has been called the "Castle of the Angel."[11] The successful procession by Pope Gregory the Great, followed by the equally successful Sebastian procession in A.D. 683, established the tradition in Europe of staging processions to appeal to God to end plagues.

In 1348, bubonic plague was introduced into Europe by Italian traders returning from the Black Sea. The first pass of the disease through Europe has come to be known as the Black Death. Twenty-five percent of Europe's population eventually died of the plague. The largest cities, particularly trading centers, were affected early and severely. Initially, the catastrophe was attributed to the poisoning of the wells by Jews. Confessions were extracted from the Jews through torture. In what is now eastern France and Switzerland, all Jews over the age of five were burned alive.[12]

The Black Death crossed and recrossed Europe, leaving the population devastated and demoralized.[13] Rich or poor, pious or sinner, young or old, anyone might die. People literally could be well in the morning and dead by dark, although most patients succumbed after a week of agony. The death carts rolled through the streets at dawn picking up the newly dead and taking the bodies to a common pit for disposal where the bodies were buried without any religious ceremony, since most priests had died or had fled into the countryside.[14] The bells tolled constantly to mark the deaths until the authorities ordered them silenced, for their constant ringing depressed those still living.[15]

The church, Roman and Catholic, had an explanation for this disease catastrophe. It must surely be God's wrath upon humankind for its many sins. In some parts of Europe, barefoot processions of penitents proceeded from village to village, saying and singing their prayers to God. In some villages and towns, it seemed to work, and the plague moved elsewhere. But, despite their newfound piety, other towns that had seemed completely spared were suddenly devastated.

The processions became longer, formalized and bloody. People beat themselves with whips in imitation of the scourging of Christ and his journey to the cross. They formed brotherhoods that marched from town to town, performing their rites of self-flagellation and singing hymns of praise. Thus were born the Flagellant Christian Brotherhoods. They sought to appease the wrath of God upon his children by imitating the suffering of Christ.

With so many people dying so rapidly, and so many fearing for their souls, charitable religious organizations experienced a veritable flood of donations and bequests. Most such money was used to provide succor to the poor and dying, but some was used to commission paintings, sculpture and architecture that would inspire and ennoble the human spirit. Surviving artists and scientists were well supported.[16] The Renaissance, that great outpouring of art and science that we so admire for its creativity and beauty, occurred in the midst of repeated waves of bubonic plague. To a considerable extent, the Renaissance occurred as a result of the economic, social and psychological stress generated by plague. At the time, paintings, whether hanging in churches or carried in religious processions, brought to the great mass of the people the dominant ideas of that age, for only a small elite in the population could read the written word. Paintings and sculptures told stories for the masses. Stories, in turn, taught concepts and explained ideas.

In Florence, in 1350, Giovanni del Biondo produced the earliest surviving painting of Saint Sebastian shot full of arrows (see Plate Three).[17] Although pierced with so many arrows that he resembles a porcupine tied to a post, Sebastian appears neither dead nor frightened. He was an apt symbol for courage in adversity and for hope during crisis.

Among the most beautiful works of the Renaissance is the painting of Saint Sebastian by Sodoma, completed in 1528 for the Company of Saint Sebastian in Camolia (see Plate Four).[18] Sebastian appears as a handsome, nearly naked young man gazing heavenward with hope, unaware of the arrow through his neck. This canvas is also a plague banner, and so is painted on both sides. On the reverse are the brethren of the Company with several other saints. It was made to be carried through the streets in times of pestilence to rally the people in a procession like that of Pope Gregory the Great.

While many saints were invoked to intercede on the behalf of those threatened by plague, Saint Sebastian became the most popular and presumably the most powerful. During the plague of 1464 in San Gimignano, near Sienna, Benozzo Gozzoli depicted the ability of Saint Sebastian to frustrate God's will (see Plate Five).[19] God, portrayed as a bearded elderly man assisted by angels, drops the arrows of pestilence onto the people of San Gimignano, identified by the contemporary skyline of their town. Saint Sebastian stands with outspread cape, blocking the rain of arrows and saving the people. During the same plague, Bonfigli painted Mary, the mother of Jesus, protecting the townspeople of Perugia with her cape (see Plate Six).[20] The enormous figure of Mary dominates the canvas, conveying the intense drive of a mother to protect her children, even when they deserve punishment. Above, an almost incidental figure of Jesus wields the arrows of pestilence while the Archangel Michael holds the drawn sword of judgment on the right and the sheathed sword of mercy on the left. Below and outside the walls of Perugia, bat-winged death, armed with bow and arrows, is slain by an angel. This suggests that even if one dies of the plague, the sting of death has been taken away by the intercession of Mary.

That Mary, the earthly mother of Jesus, could and would protect the people from the wrath of God became a popular belief. This was visually expressed as Mary protecting people with her cloak and is called a "Misericordia della Madonna" figure.[21] Originally associated only with pestilence, the image soon came to represent Mary's protection from any of the punishments or torments sent by God. This was a time of rapid growth in the cult of Mary. With the people believing that Jesus killed off masses of people indiscriminately for the sins of society, Mary offered compassion and forgiveness. Kings, bishops and city princes asked God to spare their realms and promised various gifts if God would relent from destroying them. Their vows were as grand as their positions, and plague churches were erected all over Europe. The Karlkirche, in Vienna, fulfilled the vow of the Hapsburg Emperor, Charles V, to build a great church if God would lift the plague of 1712.[22] When the plague ended, Charles V believed it was as a result of those promises, and, true to his word, he built the church, raising the money by imposing a new tax on his people.

Frequently visited by plague, Venice, the wealthiest trading city of the Renaissance, built five plague churches from the fifteenth to the seventeenth century, and the painters Titian, Veronese and Tintoretto, among others, filled them with art designed to inspire good works in time of disaster.[23] Thus, the Roman Catholic Church provided a bridge between humans and God across the chasm of plague, and the artists of that time explained its workings to the people, their art serving as a record of human experience.

Though often neglected by historians, epidemic disease has been a powerful force in the shaping of ideas and of social institutions. As a major influence on society, epidemics and their effects have been frequent subjects for artists (see Plates Seven, Eight, Nine and Ten). It is no accident of history that our contemporary artistic community is active in the AIDS epidemic. Artists reflect the issues facing a society. Now, as during the Renaissance, artists educate the public about the threat of an epidemic (see Plates Eleven, Twelve and Thirteen). Physicians, lecturing about viral particles and safer sex, have only a slight influence on the behavior of people. Using paint, music, words or film, artists tell the story of disease in a way that intimately relates it to the lives of all the people and educates society. It is largely through the work of the artistic community that a society comes to understand its problems and their solutions. This will be true also with AIDS, the newest in a long series of epidemics.

Notes

1. Immanuel Jakobovits, *Jewish Medical Ethics: A Comparative and Historical Study of the Jewish Religious Attitude to Medicine and Its Practice* (New York: Bloch Publishing, 1959), 1–4 and 96–98.

2. Arturo Castiglioni, *Christian Dogmatic Medicine* (New York: Knoff, 1947).

3. Raymond Crawfurd, *Plague and Pestilence in Literature and Art* (Oxford: Clarendon Press, 1914), 74.

4. Arturo Castiglioni, "The Political Decadence of the Empire: The Great Epidemics," *A History of Medicine* (New York: Knoff, 1947), 242–44.

5. His importance as a plague figure was established in *The Golden Legend of Jacobus de Voragine*, G. Ryan and H. Ripperger, trans. (New York: Aron Press, 1969), 104–10.

6. E. Boyd, *Popular Art of Spanish New Mexico* (Santa Fe, New Mexico: Museum of New Mexico Press, 1974), 462–66 for a discussion of the Death Cart. See page 413 for a picture of Dona Sebastiana, la Muerte or Death by Jose B. Ortega.

7. Donald Attwater and Herbert Thurston, eds. *Butler's Lives of the Saints*, vol. 1 (New York: P. J. Kenedy and Sons, 1956), 128–30.

8. For the earliest material on St. Sebastian see *Guide to the Basilica and the Catacomb of Saint Sebastian* S.I. 2nd ed., Antonio Ferrua (Vatican City, Pontifical Commission of Sacred Archaeology, 1983).

9. The description of the plague in A.D. 680 in Italy, at that time ruled by the Lombards with their capital at Pavia, is given in the *History of the Lombards*, book 6, Paul the Deacon, William D. Foulke, trans. (Philadelphia, University of Pennsylvania Press, 1907 and 1974), 254–55.

10. The description of the Plague of Justinian, A.D. 542–43, occurs in the *History of the Wars, Secret History and Buildings*, Procopius, Averil

Cameron, trans. (New York: Twayne Publishers, 1967). (The actual description is in the *History of the Wars*, book 2, 115–24.)

11. Marica Mercalli, "The Angel of the Castle: Its Iconography, Its Significance," *The Angel and Rome* (Rome: Fratelli Palombi, 1987), 67–93.

12. J. F. C. Heckler, *The Epidemics of the Middle Ages* (London: I. G. Woodfall, 1844). (In the Appendix see "Examination of the Jews Accused of Poisoning the Wells, pages 70–74.)

13. John Hatcher, *Plague, Population and the English Economy 1348–1530* (New York: MacMillan, 1977), 21–26.

14. Phillip Ziegler, *The Black Death* (New York: Penguin Books, 1970), 45–51, 127–29. And *The Plague and the Fire, London: 1665/1666*, James Leasor (New York: McGraw-Hill, 1961), 136–38.

15. Robert S. Gottfried, *The Black Death, Natural and Human Disaster in Medieval Europe* (London: Robert Hale, 1983), 69–72.

16. Millard Meiss, *Painting in Florence and Sienna after the Black Death: the Arts, Religion and Society in the mid-fourteenth Century* (New York: Harper and Row, 1964), 78–80.

17. *Martyrdom of Saint Sebastian* by Giovanni del Biondo is in the Museo dell'Opera del Duomo in Florence, Italy.

18. *Saint Sebastian* by Sodoma painted in 1528. It is in the Galleria Palatina, Palazzo Pitti in Florence, Italy.

19. *Saint Sebastian Protecting the Devoted from the Plague* (1464) by Benozzo Gozzoli is in the Church of San Agostino in San Gimignano, Italy.

20. The painting by Bonfigli, completed in 1464, is presently in a storeroom in the convent attached to the ruined Church of San Francesco del Prato in Perugia, Italy.

21. Crawfurd, *Plague and Pestilence in Literature and Art*, 107.

22. The Karlkirche was built in 1717 in thanksgiving for the end of what was to be the last sweep of bubonic plague in Europe. The great

columns flanking the church celebrate the work of San Carlo Borromeo, Bishop of Milan during the Plague of 1630, who cared for the sick and dying with his own hands, inspiring the people to do the same.

23. The plague churches in Venice, that is the churches built in an effort to induce God to lift a plague or in thanksgiving that a plague had ended, are the Church of San Giobbe (1462–71), the Church of San Rocco (1485–90), the Church of San Sebastian (1506–1518), the Church of the Redentore (1577) and the Church of Santa Maria della Salute (1632).

Chapter 3

Lenti Viruses and Cultural Organization

THE DISEASE CAUSED BY HIV INFECTION, AIDS, was first described in the United States in 1981.[1] The causative agent, HIV, was identified by Luc Montagnier and his colleagues at the Pasteur Institute in Paris in 1983.[2] Within months they recognized that it was a lenti virus from its similarity to the horse lenti virus, EIAV.[3] A test for the antibody to the virus, indicating infection, was developed in 1985.[4]

HIV, the infectious agent causing AIDS, is a member of a family of viruses called the lenti viruses.[5] Lenti is the Latin word for "slow." They were given this name because of the long time between initial infection and overt illness. Other members of this viral family infect sheep, goats, horses, cattle, cats and our fellow primates, monkeys. HIV has many characteristics in common with the other lenti viruses, and by examining characteristics of the family, we can better understand the behavior of HIV and more accurately predict its effect on the human population.[6]

The study of the lenti viruses began with swamp fever, a disease of horses, first described in 1843 in France.[7] Initial efforts to identify the causative agent were not successful. Swamp fever did not begin to yield its secrets until 1904 when it was demonstrated to be a virus—in fact, one of the first viruses to be identified. It has come to be called Equine Infectious Anemia Virus, EIAV.[8]

The EIAV infection of horses is characterized by an initial flulike illness frequently followed by recurrent episodes of fever and anemia. Most infected horses survive the illness and then appear fit, living a normal or near normal life span, but are always subject to recurrences if stressed. EIAV appears to be primarily transmitted by secretions from the lungs of sick horses, sexual intercourse and in recent times, the use of contaminated needles and syringes.

The effort to make a vaccine for the horse to prevent swamp fever began with studies in the second half of the last century. Discoveries came slowly. Until 1904, no one was able to identify the microorganism causing the disease. A culture of EIAV proved impossible to grow in anything except a horse, and a horse is an unwieldy experimental animal. Eventually, a blood test to detect the presence of antibodies against the virus was developed. This allowed easy identification of infected horses, but neither an effective treatment nor an effective vaccine followed.

It was in Iceland, where the sheep industry was devastated by an epidemic inadvertently imported from Germany in the 1930s, that the lenti viruses were first more specifically isolated and characterized. The disease in sheep, called visna, was manifested as a progressive breathlessness ending in death from pneumonia or slow paralysis and dementia. Once ill, the animal died within two years. The disease was difficult to control because many sheep did not become overtly ill for years and were difficult to identify.[9]

The problem of obtaining large amounts of pure lenti virus was finally solved in 1960 by the Icelandic scientist, Bjorn Sigurdsson, and his colleagues when they grew visna virus in sheep brain cells in tissue culture.[10] In rapid succession, the other known lenti viruses were also grown in tissue culture.[11] This enabled research efforts to move much faster. However, despite this breakthrough thirty years ago, we still do not have a useful vaccine against any lenti virus, and we still do not have an effective treatment for any of the lenti virus infections.

Macaques, an Asian monkey species, began dying in research colonies in the United States during the 1970s of a disease that we now realize was caused by a lenti virus. It was subsequently named Simian Immunodeficiency Virus, SIV.[12] Its distribution in monkeys is not uniform. Among monkeys recently caught in the wild, those from Africa appear to have lenti virus infections, but not those from Asia or the Americas.

Macaques dying of SIV are analogous to the Icelandic sheep that were killed by the visna virus. The Macaques have not had experience with SIV and are not biologically adapted to it. The sheep and monkey experience illustrates that benign infections in biologically experienced animal species may be deadly in newly infected naïve species. This is the same phenomenon that caused the massive die-off of Native Americans when they were initially exposed to the Old World disease pool by the Europeans who followed Columbus.

Lenti virus infections are different from most other viral infections.[13] In the process of their evolutionary development, the lenti viruses exploited techniques to avoid control by mammals' immune systems. Instead of rapidly recognizing the invasion by a lenti virus, the immune system may take many weeks to respond. Once antibodies are finally made, they may slow the infection, but do not stop it.[14] The virus remains active in the face of a good antibody response. The virus continues to be reproduced and to infect new cells. If the mammal tests positive for antibodies to the lenti virus, the mammal is not immune. A positive test for antibodies just means that the mammal has an active lenti virus infection.[15]

Since the lenti virus cannot be killed by the immune system, it follows that lenti virus infections are active for the life of the infected mammal, however long or short that may be. As the virus infects new cells, some die and some do not function properly. When this happens to a large enough number of cells, the mammal becomes ill. If it happens to an even larger number of cells, the mammal dies.

In all lenti virus–infected mammalian species, including Homo sapiens, there is great variability in the disease course among individuals. This is probably the result of variations in individual resistance of the host mammal, in lethality of different strains of the virus, and in environmental stresses on the host.[16]

The occurrence of an epidemic involves more than just a germ and a large group of hosts. Historically, pestilence has been the faithful companion of war and famine. War stirs the population, assuring that everyone will be exposed to whatever diseases exist in the region. Famine forces the bodies of the starving to abandon defense and to expend all available energy on maintaining the essential functions of life. War and famine sorely compromise the resistance of both the community and the individuals, giving disease an opportunity to overwhelm the population.

Once considered a jewel of the British Empire, Uganda, beginning in 1971, was afflicted by the chaos of civil war. Tribal rivalries and the vicious plundering of the country by the tyrant, Idi Amin, destroyed its cities and farms and left its people shattered and exhausted. War and famine were followed by their traditional companion, pestilence.[17]

Although some men and women began to progressively lose weight, become skeletal and then die, little notice was taken in the greater tragedy of the disintegrating nation. It happened frequently enough, however, to acquire a local name, "Slim Disease." That simple name described the main symptom, progressive, irreversible weight loss until weakness led to death. We have since discovered that Slim Disease is a manifestation of AIDS.[18] Uganda, we now know, experiences the highest HIV infection rate of any country in the world, some 10 to 20 percent of the entire adult population.[19]

HIV probably crossed over to humans in the middle years of this century in Uganda, along the western shore of Lake Victoria, the largest lake in Africa, or just to the west in the drainage of the Congo River. The source of the crossover was most likely SIV, from our closest mammalian relative, the monkey. The transfer probably occurred in an isolated rural area, then spread slowly from one village to another, never attracting attention to itself as a significant disease. It eventually adapted genetically to humans, so that by the time it burst forth in America as a new disease, it was quite distinct from the monkey virus that probably was its parent.[20]

It is not possible to know the exact circumstances of the lenti virus crossover into humans. It may have been from a scratch, a bite or the blood of a dying monkey spilled into an open cut. We do know that several kinds of monkeys were a food source in the area, so contact between humans and monkeys regularly occurred. Somehow, SIV was introduced into a human and was able to initiate an infection. By observing the rate of mutation of HIV, we can calculate how long it would have taken HIV to have developed from SIV. Those calculations suggest that HIV may be only forty years old, though it could be as much as several hundred years old.[21]

There have been some other suggestions for paternity of the human lenti viruses.[22] EIAV, the lenti virus in horses, and visna, the lenti virus in sheep, are the leading candidates.

The evidence, however, best supports an origin in Central Africa, where the earliest human blood found to contain antibodies to HIV was located. The greatest number of cases of AIDS are in Central Africa, and the greatest percentage of population infected with HIV is in Central Africa. Most early documented cases of AIDS occurred in individuals who had worked or traveled in Central Africa.[23]

In efforts to control the epidemic, however, points of origin are probably irrelevant. There has been an unfortunate propensity to blame Africa and Africans for the epidemic. That is absurd. The natural process by which diseases rise and fall gave us these human lenti viruses, not the people of Africa. Blaming the Africans for AIDS is as absurd as blaming the Jews for the Black Death.

Humans and HIV have had relatively little time to adapt to each other biologically. Reproduction of the virus so upsets the normal workings of the human body that the death rate will probably exceed 90 percent and may go above 99 percent. AIDS is thus the most lethal disease epidemic to strike humankind in recorded history. The slow onset of illness following infection, averaging some nine years, disguises the extraordinarily deadly nature of the epidemic.[24]

HIV, the human-hosted lenti virus, slowly made its way from person to person and village to village, spread by heterosexual intercourse, a highly reliable method of transmission, as humans are by nature not monogamous.[25] If humans were monogamous and mated for life, there probably would be no venereal diseases of any kind, as there could be no chain of infection. Many microorganisms exploit the human propensity to have more than one sexual partner during a lifetime, making human sexuality a formidable means of disease transmission.

A virus isn't alive in the usual sense. It is just a packet of instructions. It doesn't have metabolism. It doesn't move. It doesn't reproduce. It doesn't even infect. The right kind of cell must come along and ingest it. The unwary cell then reads the instructions of the virus and begins to use them. Following the instructions of the virus, the cell makes new viral parts, assembles them and disseminates them. The cell's normal functions are impaired by this new job of making viruses, and the cell may die.

In most living organisms, the genetic instructions are in the form of DNA, long chains of organic molecules that are the building blocks of genes. These direct the making of proteins, the interactions and workings of which we call life. Most viruses are packages of genetic instructions in the form of DNA.

HIV is different. HIV is a package of instructions in the form of RNA.[26] The infected cell cannot directly read the instructions in the form of RNA. The HIV instructions must be converted from RNA to DNA by an enzyme carried by the virus, using building materials and energy supplied by the cell. Once a DNA copy of the RNA has been made, the cell can then read the instructions of the virus. Because the first step in viral infection is a backward step from RNA to DNA, HIV is called a retrovirus. This RNA to DNA step has a high error rate and no correction mechanism, so the HIV mutation rate is extremely high.

After conversion, the DNA form of the HIV instructions is incorporated into the cell's own genetic material. The virus is now an aspect of the infected cell. The virus and the cell are one, and the only way to cure the infected person is to eliminate all of the HIV-infected cells. Because HIV infects cells in the brain, kidneys, skin and intestines as well as in the blood, it is not feasible to kill all of the infected cells. It is unlikely, then, that a cure can ever be found. Our best hope is to develop a treatment that causes the HIV-infected cells to stop making new virus particles. That implies a lifelong treatment for HIV infection.

Half of those infected with HIV have developed AIDS or have died of AIDS by the tenth year of infection.[27] Some people will probably live fifteen or twenty years with the infection before they develop AIDS. A few may never develop AIDS. Some will develop AIDS after only a year or two of infection. The rapidity of the onset of AIDS in an HIV-infected individual is probably dependent on the size of the infecting dose, the strain of the virus and the natural resistance of the person.

Infection with HIV begins when the viral particles enter the body and are taken up by cells. Within days to weeks, for reasons that remain obscure, the infected cells may begin to massively produce the virus. It is then present in large numbers in the blood and in the fluids derived from blood, vaginal fluids, semen and breast milk. This high viral blood level lasts a few days to a few weeks, and the person experiences a flulike illness.[28] Infrequently, an infected person will progress immediately to AIDS.[29]

Whether or not people newly infected with HIV get a flulike illness, most of them will produce enough virus to provoke an antibody response against the virus. It is this antibody response that we measure with a blood test to discover the HIV infection.[30]

A small percentage of HIV-infected people do not make enough virus to provoke antibody production, or for unknown reasons, they do not produce antibodies even when virus is present in adequate amounts. These people test negative.[31] But they can transmit the virus through blood transfusions or blood products.[32] They are probably not making enough virus to be infectious through sexual intercourse.[33]

Most people, after producing enough virus to provoke antibody production, enter a long period during which they feel fine and are unaware of their infection.[34] Viral replication is probably occurring rapidly in the lymphatic system, but the viral load in the blood is low. During this time the person's fluids are not very infectious. Hundreds or even thousands of episodes of sexual intercourse with such a person would probably not transmit the virus. Eventually, the viral load increases in the blood and the person becomes more infectious. [35] Then, within a year or two, the person begins to experience medical problems and acquires the diagnosis of AIDS. Meaningful studies of the transmission of HIV must take into account the degree of infectiousness.[36] Infectiousness varies according to the stage of illness—early stage, high infectiousness for a few weeks; middle stage, low infectiousness for years; and late stage, high infectiousness falling to low as death approaches.[37]

Three drugs appear to be modestly effective in treating HIV disease. They are AZT , ddI and ddC.[38] They are all artificial building blocks for the making of DNA.[39] All of them work by interfering with the transcription of RNA into DNA, which prevents the infection of new cells. They do not interfere with virus production in already-infected cells, so HIV is not eliminated from the patient. The old HIV-infected cells continue to make new HIV particles in the presence of these drugs, but the infection of new cells is partially blocked. Therefore, these drugs do not cure the patient, but they do slow down the progression of the disease, and probably make the patient less infectious.

HIV infection itself lowers resistance to disease-causing microorganisms because it infects and lives in the defense system of the body. The defense system eventually becomes so damaged by HIV that disease may be caused by microorganisms that are usually harmless. We call these unusual diseases opportunistic infections.[40] The pneumocystis carinii microorganism, a type of yeast, is not normally a disease-causing microorganism. It has long been known to medical science as causing pneumonia in malnourished children in refugee camps.[41] Starvation so reduces their resistance that pneumocystis can infect them and cause overt disease. Today, pneumocystis pneumonia is familiar to us as a disease of AIDS patients. It is an opportunistic infection that occurs because the immune system is suppressed by HIV. Pneumonia caused by pneumocystis eventually occurs in 80 percent of AIDS patients in North America.[42]

The ordinary disease-causing microorganisms can also infect, sicken and kill HIV-infected patients. They readily develop pneumonia, tuberculosis, syphilis, hepatitis B, herpes and chicken pox.[43] The AIDS patients provide a potential reservoir for these infectious diseases. While healthy people are at no risk of acquiring HIV from casual contact with AIDS patients, they may be at risk for acquiring hepatitis B and tuberculosis. These diseases can be severe and life threatening, even in a person with a normal immune system. The HIV epidemic is creating secondary epidemics of tuberculosis and other infectious diseases among non-HIV-infected persons.

We are already seeing an upsurge of active tuberculosis in HIV-infected IV heroin addicts in New York City, in New Jersey and in Miami.[44] Several outbreaks of tuberculosis have occurred in medical personnel and prison guards serving this patient population. As these HIV- and tuberculosis-infected individuals share elevators and subways and other confined spaces with other people, some of those people will become infected with tuberculosis.

At present, the problem is a small one because there are so few HIV-infected people. But, as the HIV epidemic grows, the phenomenon of secondary epidemics will become increasingly troublesome.[45] Casual contacts at no risk of acquiring HIV will be at risk of acquiring hepatitis B or tuberculosis.

A person with tuberculosis is dramatically helped by antibiotics, which slow down and hinder the tuberculosis microorganisms so effectively that a person's own defense system is able to bring the infection under control. What if the person's immune system is damaged by HIV? The antibiotics slow down and hinder the tuberculosis, but the damaged immune system is not able to bring it under control.[46] When the antibiotic is stopped, the tuberculosis reactivates. The antibiotic must be given for the rest of the patient's life.[47] As the tuberculosis bacilli continue to be bathed in antibiotic, the less resistant ones die and the most resistant ones reproduce. Gradually, the strain of tuberculosis becomes increasingly resistant to the antibiotic until, finally, the antibiotic is useless against that strain. To hold the tuberculosis in check, a new and different antibiotic must then be given. The cycle begins again. This problem of the development of antibiotic resistance by disease microorganisms has been known for many years. It was a problem before the arrival of HIV. We use techniques like simultaneous multiple drug therapy to inhibit the development of resistant strains of bacteria. While this is a clever strategy, it only slows down the development of resistant strains. It does not *prevent* the development of resistant strains. We have long been in a race to develop new antibiotics before our old ones become ineffective.[48]

Now we face HIV. Our patients may not clear ordinary infections even with the help of antibiotics.[49] In some circumstances, we must indefinitely use antibiotics to suppress the infection. We know that this indefinite use of antibiotics will accelerate the development of antibiotic resistance in disease microorganisms.

Poverty is the companion of disease. Premature births, unwanted pregnancies, mental retardation, drug addiction, alcoholism, broken homes, child abandonment and criminal behavior all afflict the poor in disproportionate numbers. Those living in poverty have a poor diet, poor housing, poor medical care and often lack family structure. These factors degrade the general level of health, making poor people more vulnerable to disease. Overcrowding assures that exposure to infectious, disease-causing microorganisms will occur frequently. Compromised resistance to infectious disease, individually and in a community sense, accompanies poverty. Invasion of the poor communities by disease microorganisms is relatively easy. Tuberculosis, syphilis, gonorrhea, measles, polio, meningitis and hepatitis are all found in greatest abundance among the poor.

The life processes of the lenti viruses, including HIV, enhance their transmission and survival in small groups of animals. Humans would have been invaded by our lenti virus, HIV, only gradually and over many generations if we still lived under the hunter-gatherer form of social organization. Small groups with infrequent contact would have spread HIV through the human population very slowly. It is the functioning of modern human society, not some unique feature of our human biology, that has disseminated HIV so rapidly. The way we have organized ourselves as a culture has made us uniquely vulnerable to a sudden, severe, socially disruptive invasion by HIV.

Biology determines that an infection can occur. Culture determines who is exposed, when they are exposed and how rapidly the disease microorganism is disseminated. The important influence of the modern, crowded, chaotic and poverty-stricken city on transmission rates of HIV can be seen in the difference in the spread of HIV in rural Zaire and in Kinshasa, the rapidly growing capital of Zaire. In isolated rural northwestern Zaire, in Equateur Province, the infection rate for HIV in 1976 was 0.8 percent and in 1986 was the same.[50] In Kinshasa, the infection rate for HIV had risen to about 5 percent by 1986.[51] The modern city creates a unique setting for rapid spread of HIV through the human population.

The way we have organized ourselves as a culture imposes a set of risks on men and women that makes some of them extremely vulnerable to HIV infection. The lenti virus epidemics in sheep and goats resulted from high group risks, not high-risk individual behavior. This suggests that the HIV epidemic in humans should be controllable with thoughtful social policies that lower group risks by conscious decision if we have the requisite political will. This should be effective even in the absence of cooperation from individuals engaging in high-risk behaviors. We should be able to change our culture in ways that will protect entire segments of the population. With this approach, the HIV epidemic should be controllable even in the absence of an effective vaccine and curative treatment.

The HIV epidemic creates many costs for our society that are not direct and not obvious. Among these costs will be the increase in the disease burden in the non-HIV-infected portion of the population and an increase in disease resistance to antibiotics, making treatment of ordinary infections less effective and more expensive. HIV has the effect of lowering the resistance of our entire society to infectious diseases.

None of us can escape the disease consequences of the HIV epidemic. Resistance to disease is dependent on the health of every individual in our community. When our neighbor is ill, our health is at risk. If we allow HIV to infect a significant percentage of any segment of our population, everyone in the society will be at some risk from an associated problem.

Unlike our mammalian cousins, we are not limited to biological adaptation. We are not helpless even in the absence of a curative treatment and an effective vaccine. If we adequately understand the lenti viruses, we can change our vulnerability to invasion by HIV by consciously and deliberately changing our culture.

We tend to believe that infectious diseases are conquered by medical science, forgetting that science is an *aspect* of culture, and that some infectious diseases were conquered long before we had effective science. We will not be able to stop the HIV epidemic, even with effective science, if we are unwilling to make major changes in the way we function as a society. We may not want to pay increased taxes to assist heroin and cocaine addicts and gay men. We may be unwilling to devote ourselves to the care of those whom some consider to be sinners. But, if we do not care for all the members of our society, rich and poor, gay and straight, black and white, addict and prostitute, we will suffer an immense disease burden.

It will be costly to control the HIV epidemic. It will be even more costly if we do not control it. Politics and social reform—not medicine—will determine our success.

Notes

1. M. S. Gottlieb, H. M. Schanker and R. Schroff, "Pneumocystis Carinii Pneumonia and Mucosal Candidiasis in Previously Healthy Homosexual Men," *New England Journal of Medicine*, vol. 305, no. 24 (Dec. 10, 1981): 1425–31.

J. B. Greene, H. Masur and M. A Michelis, "An Outbreak of Community-Acquired Pneumocystis Carinii Pneumonia," *New England Journal of Medicine*, vol. 305, no. 24 (Dec. 10, 1981): 1431–38.

G. S. Hammer, C. Lopez and F. P. Siegal, "Severe Acquired Immunodeficiency in Male Homosexuals, Manifested by Chronic Perianal Ulcerative Herpes Simplex Lesions," *New England Journal of Medicine*, vol. 305, no. 24 (Dec. 10, 1981): 1439–44.

2. F. Barre-Sinoussi, J. C. Chermann and F. Rey, "Isolation of a T-Lymphotropic Retrovirus from a Patient at Risk for Acquired Immune Deficiency Syndrome (AIDS)," *Science*, vol. 220, no. 4599 (May 20, 1983): 868–71.

3. F. Barre-Sinoussi, J. C. Chermann and L. Montagnier, "A New Human T-Lymphotropic Retrovirus: Characterization and Possible Role in Lymphadenopathy and Acquired Immune Deficiency Syndromes," *Human T-Cell Leukemia/Lymphoma Viruses*, R. C. Gallo, M. Essex and L. Gross, eds. (New York: Cold Spring Harbor Laboratory, 1984), 363–79.

C. Axler, C. Dauguet and L. Montagnier, "A New Type of Retrovirus Isolated from Patients Presenting with Lymphadenopathy and Acquired Immune Deficiency Syndrome: Structural and Antigenic Relatedness with Equine Infectious Anaemia Virus," *Annales de Virologie* (Institute Pasteur, 1984), 119–34.

4. J. J. Goedert, M. G. Sarngadharan and S. H. Weiss, "Screening Test for HTLV-III (AIDS Agent) Antibodies. Specificity, Sensitivity, and Applications," *Journal of the American Medical Association*, vol. 253, no. 2 (Jan. 11, 1985): 221–25.

5. C. Axler, C. Dauguet and L. Montagnier, "A New Type of Retrovirus Isolated from Patients Presenting with Lymphadenopathy and Acquired

Immune Deficiency Syndrome: Structural and Antigenic Relatedness with Equine Infectious Anemia Virus," *Annales de Virologie* (Institute Pasteur, 1984), 119–34.

R. C. Gallo, M. A. Gonda and F. Wong-Staal, "Sequence Homology and Morphologic Similarity of HTLV-III and Visna Virus, A Pathogenic Lentivirus," *Science,* vol. 227, no. 4683 (Jan. 11, 1985): 173–77.

M. J. Braun, J. E. Clements and M. A. Gonda, "Human T-Cell Lymphotropic Virus Type III Shares Sequence Homology with a Family of Pathogenic Lentiviruses," Proceedings of the National Academy of Sciences of the United States of America, vol. 83. no. 11 (June 1986): 4007–11.

6.   D. Huso, O. Narayan and M. C. Zink, "Lentiviruses of Animals Are Biological Models of the Human Immunodeficiency Viruses," *Microbial Pathogenesis,* vol. 5, no. 3 (Sept. 1988): 149–57.

M. Dawson "Lentivirus Diseases of Domesticated Animals," *Journal of Comparative Pathology,* vol. 99, no. 4 (Nov. 1988): 401–19. (This is an excellent review of the subject.)

7.   W. P. Cheevers and T. C. McGuire, "Equine Infectious Anemia Virus: Immunopathogenesis and Persistence," *Reviews of Infectious Diseases,* vol. 7, no. 1 (Jan.–Feb. 1985): 83–88.

8.   Olof Dietz and Ekkehard Wiesner, eds., A. S. Turner, trans., *Diseases of the Horse: A Handbook for Science and Practice* (New York: S. Karger, 1984), 282–87.

9.   The Story of Iceland's struggle with visna is told by one of the principles in Chapter 2, pages 17–43, "Maedi and Visna in Sheep," by P. A. Palsson in *Slow Virus Diseases of Animals and Man,* R. H. Kimberlin, ed. (North-Holland Publishing Co., 1976) Also see B. Sigurdsson, H. Grimsson, P. A. Plasson: "Maedi, a Chronic, Progressive Infection of the Sheep's Lungs," *Journal of Infectious Disease,* vol. 90, 1952, pp. 233–41. And see B. Sigurdsson, "Maedi, a Slow Progressive Pneumonia of Sheep: An Epizoological and Pathological Study," *British Veterinary Journal,* vol. 110, no. 7 (July 1954): 255–70.

H. Grissom, P. A. Plasson and B. Sigurdsson "Visna, a Demyelinating Transmissible Disease of Sheep," *Journal of Neuropathology and Experimental Neurology,* vol. 16, no. 3 (July 1957): 389–403.

P. A. Plasson, B. Sigurdsson and L. van Bogaert, "Pathology of Visna," *Acta Neuropathologica,* vol. 1 (1962), 343–62.

10. P. A. Plasson, B. Sigurdsson and H. Thormar, "Cultivation of Visna Virus in Tissue Culture," *Archiv fur die Gesamte Virusforschung,* vol. 10 (1960): 368–381.

H. Thormar, "The Growth Cycle of Visna Virus in Monolayer Cultures of Sheep Cells," *Virology,* vol. 19 (1963): 273–78.

11. K. Kobayashi, "Studies on the Cultivation of Equine Infectious Anemia Virus In Vitro. III. Propagation of the Virus in Leukocyte Culture, *Virus,* vol. 11 (1961), 249–56.

Y. Fukanaga, Y. Kono and T. Yoshino, "Growth Characteristics of Equine Infectious Anemia Virus in Horse Leukocyte Cultures," *Archiv fur die Gesamte Virusforschung,* vol. 30, no. 2 (1970): 252–56.

J. E. Clements, O. Narayan and J. D. Strandberg, "Biological Characterization of the Virus Causing Leukoencephalitis and Arthritis in Goats," *Journal of General Virology,* vol. 50, no. 1 (Sept. 1980): 69–79.

12. R. C. Desrosiers, R. D. Hunt and D. J. Ringler, "Simian Immunodeficiency Virus-Induced Meningoencephalitis: Natural History and Retrospective Study, *Annal of Neurology,* vol. 23, suppl. (1988): S101–S107.

13. R. J. Adams, D. E. Griffin and O. Narayan, "Early Immune Responses in Visna, A Slow Viral Disease of Sheep," *The Journal of Infectious Diseases,* vol. 138, no. 3 (Sept. 1978): 340–50.

14. G. Georgsson, J. R. Martin and N. Nathanson, "The Effect of Post-Infection Immunication on the Severity of Experimental Visna," *Journal of Comparative Pathology,* vol. 91, no. 2 (April 1981): 185–91.

W. M. Mitchell, D. C. Montefiori and W. E. Robinson, Jr., "Antibody-Dependent Enhancement of Human Immunodeficiency Virus Type 1 Infection," *Lancet,* vol. 1, no. 8589 (April 9, 1988) 790–94.

15. G. Kraus, R. Kurth and A. Werner, "AIDS: Animal Retrovirus Models and Vaccines," *Journal of Acquired Immune Deficiency Syndromes*, vol. 1, no. 3 (1988) 284–94.

16. L. Coggins and C. J. Issel: "Equine Infectious Anemia: Current Knowledge," *Journal of the American Veterinary Medical Association*, vol. 174, no. 7 (April 1, 1979): 727–33.

17. R. Caputo, "Uganda: Land Beyond Sorrow," *National Geographic*, vol. 173, no. 4 (April 1988): 468–91.

18. R. D. Mugerwa, D. Serwadda and N. K. Sewankambo, "Slim Disease: A New Disease in Uganda and Its Association with HTLV-III Infection," *Lancet*, vol. 2, no. 8460 (Oct. 19, 1985): 849–52.

19. J. W. Carswell, "HIV Infection in Healthy Persons in Uganda," *AIDS*, vol. 1, no. 4 (Dec. 1987): 223–27.

S. F. Berkley, S. I. Okware and R. Widy-Wirski, "Risk Factors Associated with HIV Infection in Uganda," *Journal of Infectious Diseases*, vol. 160, no. 1 (July 1989): 22–30.

J. Kellett, "Medicine in Uganda: The Impact of Prolonged War and Epidemic AIDS on Medical Care," *Canadian Medical Association Journal*, vol. 140, no. 6 (March 15, 1989): 699–701.

J. Chin, J. M. Mann and P. A. Sato, "Review of AIDS and HIV Infection: Global Epidemiology and Statistics," *AIDS* vol. 3, Suppl. (1989): S301–S307.

20. M. Essex and P. J. Kanki, "The Origins of the AIDS Virus," *Scientific American*, vol. 259, no. 4, (Oct. 1988): 64–71.

21. G. Schochetman, T. F. Smith and A. Srinivasan, "The Phylogenetic History of Immunodeficiency Viruses," *Nature*, vol. 333, no. 6173 (June 9, 1988): 573–75.

22. H. P. Katner and G. A. Pankey, "Evidence for a Euro-American Origin of Human Immunodeficiency Virus (HIV)," *Journal of the National Medical Association*, vol. 79, no. 10 (Oct. 1987): 1068–72.

P. K. Lewin, "Possible Origin of Human AIDS," *Canadian Medical Assocation Journal,* vol. 132, no. 10 (May 15, 1985): 1110.

23. I. C. Bygbjerg, "AIDS in a Danish Surgeon (Zaire, 1976)," *Lancet,* vol. 1, no. 8330 (April 23, 1983): 925.

J. L. Michaux, J. Sonnet and F. Zech, "Early AIDS Cases Originating from Zaire and Burundi (1962–1976)," *Scandinavian Journal of Infectious Diseases,* vol. 19, no. 5 (1987): 511–17.

S. S. Froland, P. Jenum, and C. F. Lindboe, "HIV-1 Infection in Norwegian Family before 1970," *Lancet,* vol. 1, no. 8598 (June 11, 1988): 1344–45.

J. Vandepitte, R. Verwilghen and P. Zachee, "AIDS and Cryptococcosis (Zaire, 1977)," *Lancet,* vol. 1, no. 8330 (April 23, 1983): 925–26.

L. D. Jewell, B. W. Mielke and E. Rogan, "A Case of Acquired Immune Deficiency Syndrome Before 1980," *Canadian Medical Association Journal,* vol. 137, no. 7 (Oct. 1, 1987): 637–38.

24. P. Bacchetti and A. R. Moss, "Natural History of HIV Infection," *AIDS,* vol. 3, no. 2. (Feb. 1989): 55–61.

25. B. N'Galy and R. W. Ryder, "Epidemiology of HIV Infection in Africa," *Journal of Acquired Immune Deficiency Syndromes,* vol. 1, no. 6 (1988): 551–58.

R. J. Biggar, "The Clinical Features of HIV Infection in Africa," *British Medical Journal,* vol. 293, no. 6560 (Dec. 6, 1986): 1453–54.

26. R. C. Gallo, "The AIDS Virus," *Scientific American,* vol. 256, no. 1 (Jan. 1987): 46–56.

W. A. Haseltine and F. Wong-Staal, "The Molecular Biology of the AIDS Virus," *Scientific American,* vol. 259, no. 4 (Oct. 1988): 52–62.

27. P. Bacchetti and A. R. Moss, "Natural History of HIV Infection," *AIDS,* vol. 3, no. 2 (Feb. 1989): 55–61.

28. J. P. Allain, A.C. Collier and R.W. Coombs, "Plasma Viremia in Immunodeficiency Virus Infection," *New England Journal of Medicine,* vol. 321, no. 24 (Dec. 14, 1989): 1626–31.

B. Blaauw, H. A. Kessler and J. Spear, "Diagnosis of Human Immunodeficiency Virus Infection in Seronegative Homosexuals Presenting

with an Acute Viral Syndrome," *Journal of the American Medical Association*, vol. 258, no. 9 (Sept. 4, 1987): 1196–99.
B. Tindall, D. A. Cooper, B. Donovan and R. Penny, "Primary Human Immunodeficiency Virus Infection, Clinical and Serologic Aspects," *Infectious Disease Clinics of North America*, vol. 2, no. 2 (June 1988): 329–41.

29. E. Dickmeis, R. Jordal, J. O. Nielsen and C. Pedersen, "Early Progression to AIDS Following Primary HIV Infection," *AIDS*, vol. 3, no. 1 (Jan. 1989): 45–47.

30. Goedert, Sarngadharan and Weiss, "Screening Test for HTLV-III (AIDS Agent) Antibodies." *Journal of the American Medical Association*, 221–25.

31. D. T. Imagawa, M. H. Lee and S. M. Wolinsky, "Human Immunodeficiency Virus Type 1 Infection in Homosexual Men Who Remain Seronegative for Prolonged Periods," *New England Journal of Medicine*, vol. 320, no. 22 (June 1, 1989) 1458–62.

32. P. D. Cumming, R. Y. Dodd, J. B. Schorr and E. L. Wallace, "Exposure of Patients to Human Immunodeficiency Virus Through the Transfusion of Blood Components that Test Antibody-Negative," *New England Journal of Medicine*, vol. 321, no. 14 (Oct. 5, 1989): 941–46.
J. E. Menitove, "The Decreasing Risk of Transfusion Associated AIDS," *New England Journal of Medicine*, vol. 321, no. 14 (Oct. 1989): 966–68.

33. F. Ensoli, A. Fernando and V. Fiorelli, "Letter re: Human Immunodeficiency Virus Type 1 Infection in Homosexual Men Who Remain Seronegative for Prolonged Periods," *New England Journal of Medicine*, vol. 321, no. 24 (Dec. 14, 1989): 1679.

34. N. C. Khan, R. R. Redfield and D. C. Wright, "Correlation of HIV Isolation Rate and Stage of Infection," Abstract THP.99. Third International Conference on AIDS, (June 1–5, 1987. Washington, D.C.), 180.

35. J. P. Allain, R. W. Coombs and A. C. Collier, "Plasma Viremia in Human Immunodeficiency Virus Infection," *New England Journal of Medicine*, vol. 321, no. 24 (Dec. 14, 1989): 1626–31.

36. M. Laga, H. Taelman and P. Van der Stuyft, "Advanced Immunodeficiency as a Risk Factor for Heterosexual Transmission of HIV," *AIDS*, vol. 3, no. 6 (June 1989): 361–66.

37. D. Baltimore and M. B. Feinberg, "HIV Revealed: Toward a Natural History of the Infection," *New England Journal of Medicine*, vol. 321, no. 24 (Dec. 14, 1989): 1673–75.

38. M. Alam, D. D. Ho and T. Moudgil, "Quantitation of Human Immunodeficiency Virus Type 1 in the Blood of Infected Persons," *New England Journal of Medicine*, vol. 321, no. 24 (Dec. 14, 1989): 1621–25.

H. Mitsuya, R. V. Thomas and R. Yarchoan, "In Vivo Activity Against HIV and Favorable Toxicity Profile of 2', 3'—dideoxyinosine," *Science*, vol. 245, no. 4916 (July 28, 1989): 412–15.

S. L. Nightingale, "Dideoxyinosine Available Under Treatment IND and Open Safety Protocol," *Journal of the American Medical Association*, vol. 262, no. 18 (Nov. 10, 1989): 2503.

39. M. S. Hirsch and J. C. Kaplan, "Antiviral Therapy," *Scientific American*, vol. 256, no. 4 (April 1987): 76–85.

40. D. S. Burke and R. R. Redfield, "HIV Infection: The Clinical Picture," *Scientific American*, vol. 259, no. 4 (Oct. 1988): 90–98.

41. "Principles and Practice of Infectious Diseases," 3rd ed., J. E. Bennett, R. G. Douglas and G. L. Mandell, eds. (New York: Churchill Livingstone, 1990), 2103.

42. S. L. Berk and A. Verghese, "Parasitic Pneumonia," *Seminars in Respiratory Infections*, vol. 3, no. 2 (June 1988): 172–78.

43. "Leads from the *MMWR*, Measles in HIV-Infected Children, United States," *Journal of the American Medical Association*, vol. 259, no. 16 (April 22–29, 1988): 2352, 2357.

S. Kinloch-de Loes, B. Radeff and J. H. Saurat, "AIDS Meets Syphilis: Changing Patterns of the Syphilitic Infection and Its Treatment," *Dermatologica*, vol. 177, no. 5 (1988): 261–64.

B. Maguire, and B. I. Truman, "Increasing Incidence of Tuberculosis in a Prison Inmate Population," *Journal of the American Medical Association*, vol. 261, no. 3 (Jan. 20, 1989): 393–97.

R. J. Rees and J. L. Turk, "AIDS and Leprosy," *Leprosy Review*, vol. 59, no. 3 (Sept. 1988): 193–94.

J. F. Delfraissy, L. Grangeot-Keros and V. Lazizi, "Reappearance of Hepatitis B Virus in Immune Patients Infected with the Human Immunodeficiency Virus Type 1," *Journal of Infectious Diseases*, vol. 158, no. 3 (Sept. 1988): 666–67.

Hammer, Lopez and Siegal, "Severe Acquired Immunodeficiency in Male Homosexuals," *New England Journal of Medicine,*1439–44.

44. T. Maniatis, R. J. McDonald and G. Sunderam, "Tuberculosis as a Manifestation of the Acquired Immunodeficiency Syndrome (AIDS)," *Journal of the American Medical Association*, vol. 256, no. 3 (July 18, 1986): 362–66.

45. Anonymous, "Tuberculosis and AIDS," Statement on AIDS and Tuberculosis, Geneva, March 1989. Global Programme on AIDS and Tuberculosis. World Health Organization in Collaboration with the International Union Against Tuberculosis and Lung Disease. *Bulletin of the International Union Against Tuberculosis and Lung Disease*, vol. 64, no. 1 (March 1989): 8–11.

46. Anonymous, "Diagnosis and Management of Mycobacterial Infection and Disease in Persons with Human Immunodeficiency Virus Infection," Centers for Disease Control. U. S. Department of Health and Human Services, *Annals of Internal Medicine*, vol. 106, no. 2 (Feb. 1987): 254–56.

47. F. M. Collins, "Mycobacterial disease, Immunosuppression, and Acquired Immunodeficiency Syndrome," *Clinical Microbiology Reviews*, vol. 2, no. 4 (Oct. 1989): 360–77.

48. M. H. Cynamon and S. P. Klemens, "New Antimycobacterial Agents," *Clinics in Chest Medicine*, vol. 10, no. 3 (Sept. 1989): 355–64.

49. M. D. Iseman, "Is Standard Chemotherapy Adequate in Tuberculosis Patients Infected with the HIV?" *American Review of Respiratory Disease,* vol. 136, no. 6 (Dec. 1987): 1326.

50. K. M. De Cock, D. N. Forthal and N. Nzilambi, "The Prevalence of Infection with Human Immunodeficiency Virus Over a 10–17 Year Period in Rural Zaire," *New England Journal of Medicine,* vol. 318, no. 5. (Feb. 4, 1988): 276–79.

51. H. Francis, J. M. Mann and T. C. Quinn, "HIV Seroprevalence Among Hospital Workers in Kinshasa, Zaire," *Journal of the American Medical Association,* vol. 256, no. 22 (Dec. 12, 1986): 3099–102.
K. Bila, B. N'Galy and R. W. Ryder, "Human Immunodeficiency Virus Infection Among Employees in an African Hospital," *New England Journal of Medicine,* vol. 319, no. 17 (Oct. 27, 1988): 1123–27.

Chapter 4

The Biology of
HIV Transmission

MOST TRANSMISSION OF HIV, viewed worldwide, has occurred through heterosexual intercourse.[1] A historical accident
introduced the virus into North America and Europe through
male homosexuals.[2] As the HIV epidemic matures in developed countries, it will become a primarily heterosexual disease.[3] This is hardly surprising, for there are no diseases specific to homosexuals.

Some communities also have uniquely low resistance
to infection by HIV. In Edinburgh, Scotland, in 1982 and 1983,
the community and the police were attempting to suppress IV
heroin use by drying up the supplies of needles and syringes
and with aggressive arrest practices. This forced the many IV

heroin addicts to use the same few available needles and syringes, and to use them over and over.[4] Resistance of the IV heroin addict population to infectious disease is always low. Opiates suppress the appetite, so drug users tend to be malnourished. Hygiene is often ignored in the struggle to acquire money for drugs. Into Edinburgh's community of heroin addicts in poor health, sharing twice daily the few needles and syringes that were available, came HIV. There was rapid infection of a group that was uniquely vulnerable to invasion by a blood-borne infectious agent.[5]

However, Edinburgh's gay community is largely free of HIV, and HIV's devastation of the IV drug community stands in stark contrast with its failure to penetrate the gay population in Edinburgh.[6] While the reasons for a community's resistance to a disease microorganism are difficult to describe, their absence is obvious. It would follow that it is not homosexuality or IV drug use that determines the HIV infection rate in these two very different communities. Rather, it is the special social circumstances of these two communities at a particular time in history that influences their HIV experience.

In an evolutionary sense, the strong impulse to achieve sexual pleasure assures the propagation of the human species. A considerable amount of the capacity of the human brain appears to be devoted to directing the behavior necessary to find, recognize, acquire and maintain sexual partners. The drive to accomplish sexual intercourse apparently is "hardwired" into our brains. Sexual drive isn't learned; it's innate. The pleasure of sex provides an adequate supply of children.

Modern cultural development and medical science now assure the survival of so many children that the greatest threat to the survival of the human species is from there being too many humans.

In addition to the risk of pregnancy and non-lethal venereal diseases, sexual pleasure now has a new burden: HIV. The young, especially, are told that they cannot trust those with whom they would share their bodies. The heterosexual and gay male youth must, at a minimum, maintain a barrier, a condom, between themselves and the ones they have sex with—or risk death. One may literally die from fulfilling the passion of love.

Women probably have less resistance to infection by venereal disease than men do, probably because of the physical differences between the sex organs of women and men. A woman's cervix and the large area of mucous membrane lining the walls of the vagina give microorganisms more opportunity to infect a woman than a man, whose only exposed mucous membrane is the opening of the urethra. The head of the penis and the skin of the shaft of the penis are rather more resistant to infection than is vaginal mucous membrane. This probably makes it somewhat easier to infect a woman with HIV than a man.[7]

However, the resistance of the vagina and the penis to infection by germs is considerable. In syphilis, the success of transmission of the disease microorganism to a sexual partner is only 30 percent, even when the disease is in the most infectious stage.[8] Thus, more than 70 percent of the time, syphilis infection does not occur—even when all of the conditions for transmission are present. In a society where there is no specific effort to control syphilis, syphilis does not infect everyone. Even in times of war and social chaos, when promiscuity increases, not everyone acquires syphilis.[9] Our bodies have numerous non-specific defense mechanisms, ranging from acid in the stomach to mucous in the nose to digestive enzymes in the saliva to the cornified cells of our skin. Almost no infectious disease can be transmitted by a single germ. The number of germs—the dose—must be large enough to tie up the appropriate non-specific defenses and still have germs left over.

Because we have many different kinds of effective and quite formidable defenses, disease-producing microorganisms have had to specialize their techniques of transmission and routes of invasion. Malaria must be injected into the tissue by a mosquito. Cholera can infect only when introduced through the mouth and into the intestines. HIV has been subject to these same kinds of defensive restrictions and pressures, and so it has developed its own particular dosage and transmission characteristics.

In the natural world—a world without blood transfusions and IV drug paraphernalia—HIV is transmitted from one human to another by sexual intercourse.[10] It is transmitted from man to woman, from woman to man and from man to man.[11] As with other venereal diseases, the probability that HIV will be transmitted from an infected person to a sexual partner depends on many variables. Infection does not always occur during sex between an infected person and an uninfected person. Only some of the time is an adequate dose of HIV in the semen or in the vaginal fluids of the infected person. Only some of the time does HIV-infected semen cause an infection when in contact with the vagina or rectum of the uninfected person.\Only occasionally do HIV-infected vaginal secretions cause an infection to take hold on the head of a penis. Probably the most crucial variable is the concentration of HIV particles in semen and in vaginal fluids. This concentration varies widely, depending on the stage of disease process in the infected person.[12]

To initiate an infection, HIV must enter the body in sufficient quantity to overcome the non-specific defenses. Once infection is established, HIV is produced vigorously, and high levels of virus are present in the blood. The patient will probably experience a flulike illness. This patient is highly infectious because there is a high viral concentration in all bodily fluids. Most forms of sexual intercourse at this stage of disease would expose a sexual partner to large amounts of virus. This flulike illness lasts a few days to a few weeks. Antibodies to HIV are not yet being made so that the ELISA blood test (a test to detect HIV antibodies, and therefore HIV infection) would not indicate infection. The viral load and the infectiousness fall sharply once the defense system of the patient swings into action and large amounts of antibodies against HIV are produced. The ELISA blood test then becomes positive. The patient recovers from the flulike illness and feels well.

At this point in the infection, the viral load in the blood and body fluids is low because HIV production is suppressed by the antibodies and the killer cells of the immune system. Sexual intercourse with the HIV-infected person at this stage of illness would probably not expose the sexual partner to an infectious dose of HIV.[13] This situation may last for many years. Studies of heterosexual transmission of HIV done on patients in this long period of low infectiousness may conclude that HIV cannot be transmitted through heterosexual intercourse. That would be a false and dangerous conclusion.[14]

At variable and unpredictable times during the long period of low-level HIV infection, there may be brief episodes of high virus production and high infectiousness. These are thought to occur when viral production temporarily eludes immune surveillance and escapes from defense-system control. These episodes may be precipitated by physical stress, and perhaps even by emotional stress. Such brief episodes of high infectiousness in humans may account for most of the HIV infections of sexual partners that occur when their HIV-positive partners are not yet overtly ill.

After many years of low-level HIV infection, the virus begins to overwhelm the patient's immune system. The general health of the patient declines. Colds last longer than normal. Infectiousness begins to rise.[15] Fever, weight loss and fungus infections of the mouth may begin. Infectiousness rises further. Now the probability of HIV transmission with any one episode of sexual intercourse is high, because the viral load in the blood, in the semen, or the vaginal fluids is high. But HIV transmission depends on the defenses of the sexual partner, too. A healthy sexual partner may fend off an HIV infection while a defensively weak sexual partner, a person with low disease resistance, may become infected.

As the HIV-infected person becomes increasingly ill and finally develops AIDS, infectiousness continues to increase. Then, as AIDS worsens and the body becomes wasted, infectiousness probably falls. The body may become so damaged that it can no longer produce many HIV particles.

Even when the HIV-infected person is most infectious, the likelihood of transmission occurring with any single act of sexual intercourse is probably low. *But any one act of sexual intercourse may transmit the virus.* It is not just viral load that determines transmission or the number of times a person has sexual intercourse. It is not an accumulated dose that results in HIV infection or just the health status of the sexual partner. It is a single sexual act when all the conditions for transmission are "just right" that results in infection.[16] Every episode of unprotected heterosexual or gay male sexual intercourse with an HIV-infected person increases the likelihood of hitting a time when conditions are "just right" for transmission.

The presence of another venereal disease enhances the likelihood of that person passing on or becoming infected with HIV. All of the venereal diseases that cause ulcers on the genitals—syphilis, chancroid and herpes—appear to increase transmission of HIV.[17] A genital ulcer is, in practical terms, a break in the defenses of the body. That alone would increase the likelihood of infection. An ulcer is also a point of inflammation where white blood cells gather. These are the cells that ingest and become infected with HIV. This makes a genital ulcer a point of easy entry or egress of HIV.

Circumcision—the surgical removal of the penis's foreskin—appears to have some protective effect against HIV infection.[18] The foreskin of the uncircumcised male, if not kept meticulously clean, is frequently the home of non-specific infections that attract white blood cells. The inflamed foreskin acts like an ulcer and increases the ease of HIV infection. Uncircumcised males are thus more likely to become infected with HIV than are circumcised males.

Kissing, even in the "Age of AIDS," is safe. Although HIV can be found in the saliva, the virus is easily defeated by the defenses of the mouth, which include enzymes and non-specific antibodies.[19] In kissing, the dose of the virus is small and the route is not efficient. Even saliva from a human bite will probably not transmit HIV.[20] Although there is one reported case of HIV transmission attributed to a human bite, it involved blood from broken-out teeth.[21] The possibility of those precise circumstances ever recurring is too small to be calculated.

Transmission of HIV by oral sex occurs rarely. Semen deposited in the mouth and vaginal fluids sucked into the mouth may provide an adequate dose of HIV for infection, but the route is improper. The enzymes in the saliva digest the virus, and stomach acid dissolves the virus. A few reported cases in the medical literature of HIV transmission between females do exist. These infections may have come about during mouth-to-vagina sex (cunnilingus).[22] There also have been a few reports of HIV transmission through oral sex between men involving placement of the penis in the mouth (fellatio), with ejaculation of semen.[23]

Most HIV-infected children have obtained the virus from their mothers.[24] About one third of the infants born to HIV-infected mothers will be infected.[25] We do not know why some of the infants are HIV-infected, but most are not. Transmission is at least partially related to the types of antibodies that the mother makes to the virus.[26] There is even a case of a set of twins in which one twin is infected and one is not.[27] There is some suggestion that the sicker a woman is with the HIV infection, the more likely that her infant will be infected.[28] This would, then, agree with other transmission data that suggests that infectiousness rises with the advance of HIV disease.[29] This variable transmission of infectious disease to the fetus is not unique to HIV. Many diseases have inexplicable variations in the way they are transmitted from mother to fetus.

HIV can be transmitted from mother to newborn infant in breast milk. This has been convincingly demonstrated in cases in which an HIV-negative mother has given birth to an HIV-negative child. Later, when the mother became infected by an HIV-contaminated blood transfusion, the nursing baby became infected, too.[30] Newborns, it seems, are susceptible to HIV infection through the intestinal tract although adults are probably not. There will probably be many cases of HIV-infected mothers nursing their HIV-negative children and not infecting them. Transmission of HIV is quite variable by most routes. There's no reason to suspect that the breast-milk route will be different.

Children infected with HIV through being born to an infected mother have a 50 percent chance of living to be nine years of age (equivalent to the third grade). Many will live long enough to reach junior high, and some will survive to attend high school. As the AIDS epidemic moves gradually into the heterosexual population, the numbers of children born to HIV-infected mothers will increase, and the number of HIV-infected children in our schools will gradually increase. For some time we thought that children infected as a result of being born to an HIV-infected mother had a short life expectancy, generally two years. However, this impression was based on identifying infected children after they became ill, biasing the data toward a short life expectancy. Now we know that HIV-infected children will have a life expectancy similar to that of adults, and that most HIV-infected children will live long enough to attend school.[31]

Transmission of the virus through blood transfusion is one exception to HIV's generally "hit or miss" approach. All blood taken from HIV-infected persons is infected. A person receiving a single transfusion of HIV-infected blood will become infected with HIV. Even when the donor is in the lowest possible state of HIV infectiousness, a single blood transfusion will cause infection. A blood transfusion is the most certain way to transmit HIV. It is much more certain than sexual intercourse. This method of transmission comes as close to 100 percent as any biological system ever can.[32] (However, someone who needs a blood transfusion should get it; the fear of HIV infection shouldn't stand in the way. The chance of receiving an HIV-infected unit of blood is extremely low compared to the chance of dying from the condition that is causing the need for a blood transfusion. The chance of survival is greatest if the blood is used.)

The level of HIV infection in the adult population of the United States and Europe is still relatively low, so the frequency of infection in donated blood is low, but the HIV epidemic is expanding.[33] There is a rising level of HIV infection in the population, so the pool of HIV-infected people who are not yet making the antibodies is increasing. ELISA, the current HIV test of the blood, identifies people who are making antibodies to HIV. Because it does not test for the virus directly, ELISA misses HIV-infected blood from people who are in the early stage of infection (the first six to ten weeks) and are not yet making antibodies.[34] This is causing the blood supply for transfusions to become less safe, despite the blood-testing program. We do not know what percentage of HIV-infected people do not make antibodies for months or even years. We have no practical way to identify these people. The guesses are from a few percent to, at most, 20 percent.[35] All of these unidentified HIV-infected people will eventually begin to make antibodies, and so they'll eventually become identifiable as HIV infected. Only by controlling the HIV epidemic can we keep our blood supply from being a source of HIV infection. If we could stop new HIV infections from occurring in this country, within a few years this troublesome HIV-infected, antibody-negative

population would disappear. Only enlightened political decisions promoting social policies that will stem the HIV epidemic
everywhere in the population can make our blood supply safe.
HIV will continue to enter the veins of middle-class Americans
in gleaming high-tech hospitals if HIV is allowed to run rampant in the gay male and IV-drug-using populations, and in
big city ghettos. HIV will leak into the middle class by a number of routes, among them blood transfusions, so long as HIV
is uncontrolled in any group. To protect ourselves, we must
care for each other.

HIV exists as an epidemic disease because of the way
we organize ourselves as a culture, not because individuals go
and get the disease microorganism through high-risk behavior. Evolutionary biology gives us the disease microorganism.
Cultural organization determines how many people and which
people will be infected. Because HIV in America is concentrated in male homosexuals and impoverished blacks, many
people mistakenly believe that white, heterosexual, middle-
class America is somehow immune to HIV. That is a false and
dangerous belief. White, heterosexual, middle-class America
will acquire HIV infection more slowly than have gay men and
blacks, but just as certainly. Syphilis provides a guide to what
we will experience with HIV.

Early in this century, before the discovery of penicillin,
it is thought that syphilis infected about 10 percent of the adult
population of Europe and America.[36] While America and Europe have changed in many ways over the last ninety years,
our social structure and our sexual relationships are pretty

much the same. It is reasonable to suppose that rates of HIV infection in Europe and America will eventually be of the same magnitude as those of pre-penicillin syphilis.

Syphilis is extremely sensitive to penicillin. But even though penicillin is cheap, easily administered and effective against syphilis, syphilis continues to be a problem in the First World. Difficulty in controlling syphilis, even when there is a simple, inexpensive, curative treatment, bodes ill for efforts to control HIV.

Although we cannot directly compare the rates of infection of syphilis and HIV because their biology is so different, they both rely on sexual intercourse as their primary mode of transmission, and both are long illnesses with variable periods of infectiousness. The rates of syphilis cases varied widely in different populations prior to the introduction of penicillin. We know that the variations were not dependent upon variations in the virulence of the syphilis microorganism, so human cultural factors had to account for the difference.

In a classic work on syphilis in 1937, *Shadow on the Land,* Thomas Parran, then the U.S. surgeon general, pointed to the success of the Danes and the Swedes in controlling syphilis.[37] In 1919, Sweden had 5,976 cases of syphilis and in 1933 only 431.[38] These reductions in syphilis cases took place before the introduction of penicillin. In 1935, upper New York State with a population the same size as Sweden had 21,984 cases of syphilis.[39]

Taking the approach that syphilis was a public health problem involving the entire society, the Danes and Swedes provided free testing, free medicine, free treatment, free hospitalization and social support. They had explicit sexual education campaigns.[40] They also had involuntary testing and treatment for the few people who refused to cooperate.[41] Prostitution was outlawed. In Sweden there was mandatory tracing of sexual contacts.[42] Although raising questions about individual rights and privacy, this vigorous social program, aided by a moderately effective drug, Arsphenamine, reduced syphilis to a minor health problem.

In the United States, Arsphenamine was expensive, treatment was expensive, and hospitalization was expensive. Social-support programs were virtually nonexistent. Education was limited and emphasized abstinence. Syphilis was presented as a moral problem. The United States syphilis rates were five to twenty times higher than the Danish and Swedish rates.

The moral approach to the control of venereal disease, as promulgated in the United States, assumed that the human sexual drive could be controlled or denied for years, through willpower alone. The moral approach maintained that anyone who acquired a venereal disease deserved it. The moral program for the control of syphilis was a failure.

Sweden learned from its experience with syphilis, and it is applying the same public health measures to the problem of HIV.[43] The United States is applying the same moral approach to HIV that it applied so unsuccessfully to syphilis. The outcomes of the Swedish and American approaches to HIV can be expected to mirror their respective outcomes with syphilis.

Disease microorganisms infect populations, but because individuals become ill, we consider health (absence of disease) to be an individual concern. We tend to ignore that the health of each of us is dependent upon the health of everyone in our community. If our neighbors have an infectious disease, we are likely to get it also. Likewise, if a disease is nonexistent or rare in our community then we are unlikely to get it regardless of our own personal behavior because we have no way to acquire it. The best way for the individual to stay healthy is to make sure that the entire community is healthy.

Moral judgments about innocence and guilt, victims and criminals do not help us to understand the HIV epidemic. Individual behaviors do not cause epidemics. Even high-risk individual behaviors do not cause epidemics. Evolutionary biology gives us the infectious disease microorganism, and social organization determines who will be at high risk or at low risk for infection.

A common statement about this epidemic is that "HIV does not get you. You get HIV." The implication is that if you did not engage in risky sexual behavior, you would not become infected. But what of infected children? What of blood transfusion recipients? What of HIV-infected monogamous people whose partners cheated on them? With rare exception, no one goes out and deliberately gets an HIV infection. Rather, the person engages in an activity that, in our society at this particular time in history, leads to exposure to HIV.

A disease microorganism "gets" individuals because those individuals live within a social structure that permits the disease to flourish. Gay men, IV heroin addicts, dentists, doctors, nurses and raw-oyster eaters are all likely to "get" hepatitis B in America. Hepatitis B infects 200,000, makes 10,000 very ill, and kills 5,000 American citizens each year.[44]

An effective vaccine for hepatitis B has been available in America since 1982.[45] That vaccine, widely used, could have already eliminated hepatitis B from America. But our society, through the decisions of our political leaders, has decided not to spend the money to buy that vaccine. That decision means that illness and death from hepatitis B will continue indefinitely in America. It will continue to strike hardest among those who are at highest risk. Who, then, is responsible when an IV heroin addict goes out and "gets" hepatitis B from using a dirty syringe? Who is responsible when a transfusion recipient "gets" hepatitis B? Who is responsible when a nurse "gets" hepatitis B from an accidental needle stick injury while drawing blood from a patient? (Is the nurse at fault because she made a mistake and accidentally stuck herself? Is the hospital at fault because she was involuntarily assigned to that patient?)

When politicians decided that halting hepatitis B was not worth spending the money it would take to buy the vaccine, the people who made those public health decisions permitted hepatitis B to circulate among U.S. citizens. They knew that the disease would infect thousands of citizens as they go about their ordinary lives. What, then is high-risk behavior? Living in America?

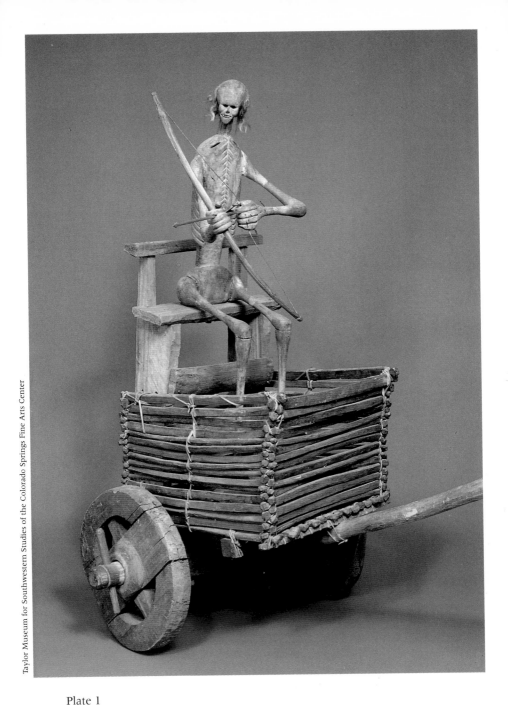

Plate 1
Death cart figure, Nasario Lopez, late nineteenth century.
St. Sebastian, who came to symbolize hope during times of epidemic disease, is shown here in this northern New Mexico Santos art figure. The details of this transformation are lost in history but are presumably related to the transport of the legend from the Old World to the New World.

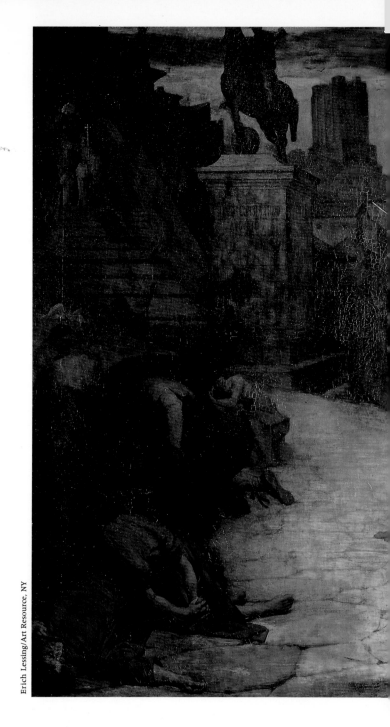

Erich Lessing/Art Resource, NY

Plate 2

The Plague in Rome, Jules-Elie Delaunay, 1869.

An angel directs the marking of the doors of those who are to die of plague in seventh-century Rome, as recounted in the history written by the eighth century

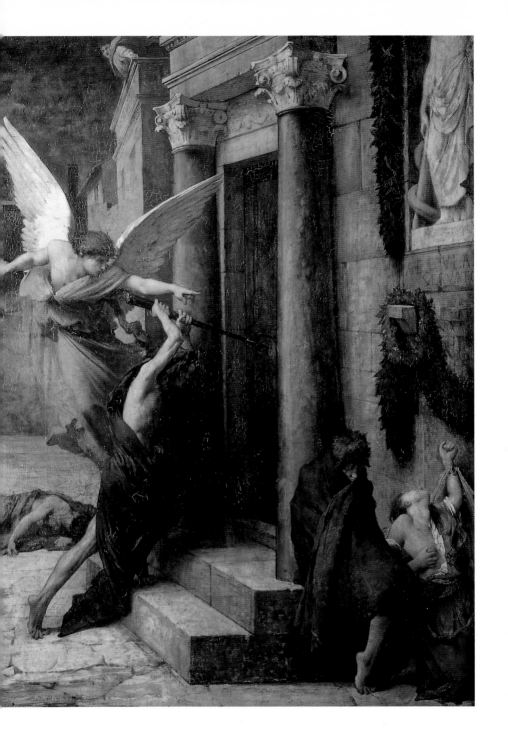

English monk, John the Deacon. Defenseless against an epidemic propagated by God's angels, Rome was saved by an appeal to St. Sebastian.

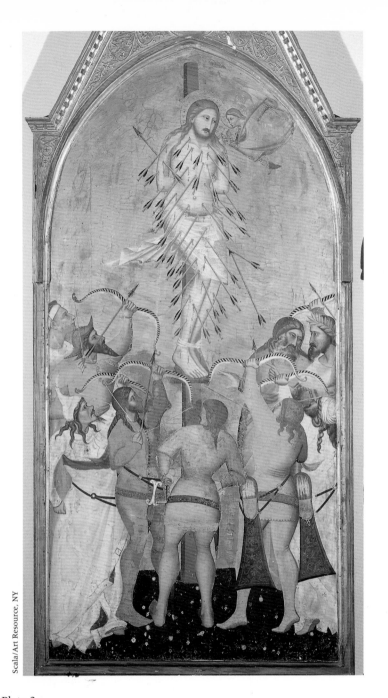

Plate 3

Martyrdom of St. Sebastian, Giovanni del Biondo, 1350.

Despite the many arrows piercing his body, St. Sebastian did not die from his wounds and was nursed back to health by Christian friends. As the arrow had been a symbol of disease since the time of the Trojan War, Sebastian came to symbolize hope and courage during times of epidemic disease.

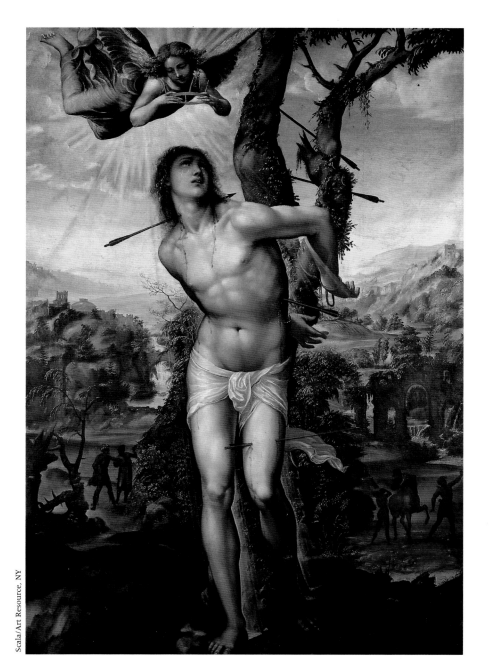

Plate 4

Saint Sebastian, Sodoma, 1528.

St. Sebastian, the "disease saint," provided an opportunity for artists to explore male beauty and physique as he was the only male saint whose iconography permitted a nearly nude portrayal. This painting appears on a double-sided plague banner, which was used in religious processions during times of plague.

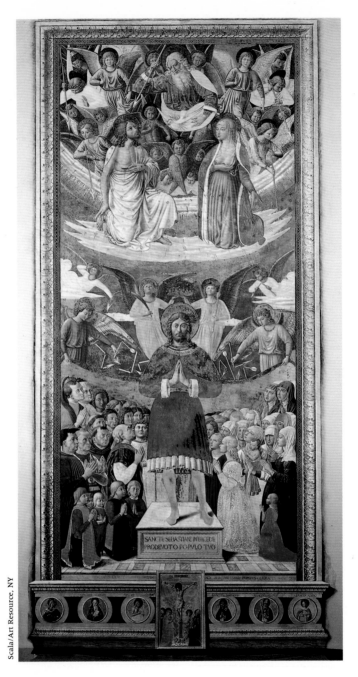

Plate 5

Saint Sebastian Protecting the Devoted from the Plague, Benozzo Gozzoli, 1464.
Produced during the plague of 1464, this representation of God and his angels
dropping arrows on the townspeople of San Gimignano vividly depicts the
belief that epidemic disease is heaven sent. St. Sebastian, with his cape out-
stretched, provides the people with some protection from the wrath of God.

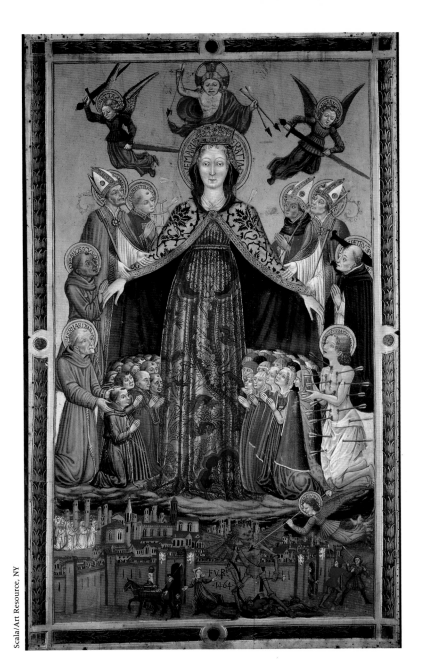

Plate 6

Misericordia della Madonna (Madonna of Mercy), Benedetto Bonfigli, 1464.
At times Mary took on the duties of St. Sebastian. In this work, produced
during the same plague as Gozzoli's painting (Plate 5), the figure of Jesus
wields the arrows of pestilence while Mary with her cape protects the people
of Perugia. Derived from the plague vision of Pope Gregory the Great, the
Archangel Michael brandishes the swords of judgment and mercy on each
side of Mary's head.

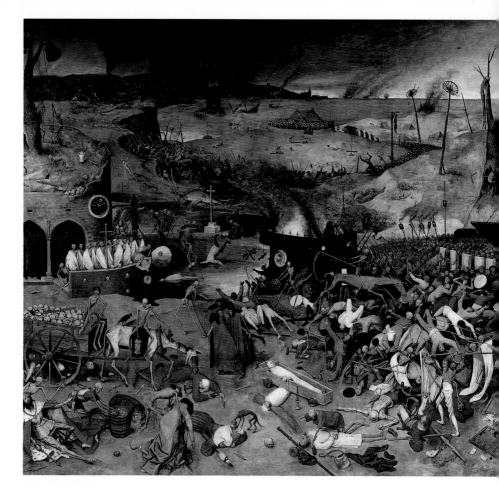

Plate 7 (above)
Triumph of Death, Pieter Brueghel (the Elder), 1556.
Beginning in 1348, plague swept back and forth through Europe, terroriz-
ing the population, inspiring the artists and molding the culture. Our present
beliefs about AIDS are, to a considerable extent, derived from our culture's
past experience with plague in Europe, symbolically depicted here in this
painting by Brueghel.

Plate 8 (opposite)
Untitled, Brent Watkinson, 1992.
In a style reminiscent of Brueghel's *Triumph of Death,* this painting addresses
our contemporary social problems with images reflecting the current epidemics of AIDS, tuberculosis, crime and environmental destruction. This work
was recently combined with Brueghel's on the cover of an issue of *Science*
magazine that details the tuberculosis/AIDS connection.

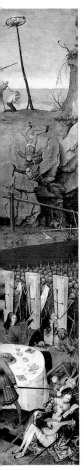

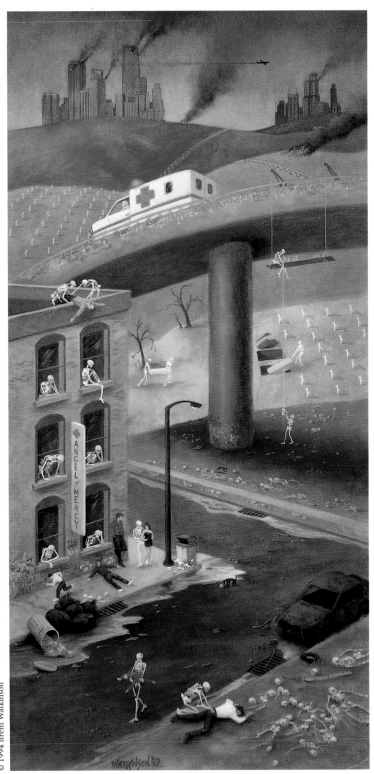

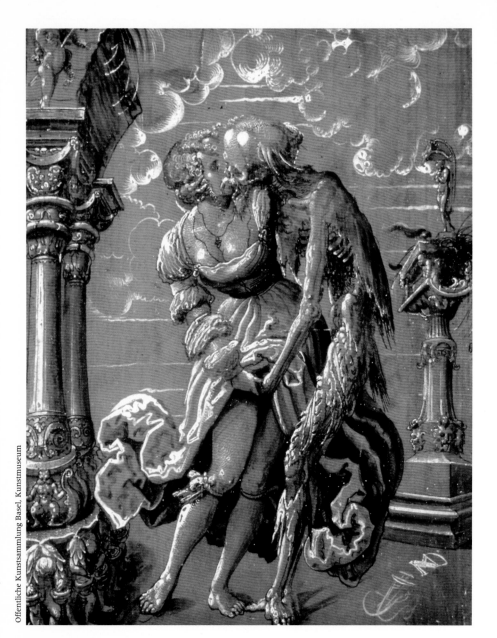

Plate 9

Der Tod als Kriegsknecht umfasst ein junges Mädchen (Death, as a soldier [war-servant], embraces a young woman), Niklaus Manuel Deutsch, 1517.

Syphilis, introduced into Europe in 1493 by the returning crew of Christopher Columbus and spread by the vagaries of war, inspired this painting symbolically pairing sex and death. Syphilis was then a deadly disease and was called the "great pox" to distinguish it from the other deadly disease with skin lesions, the "small pox."

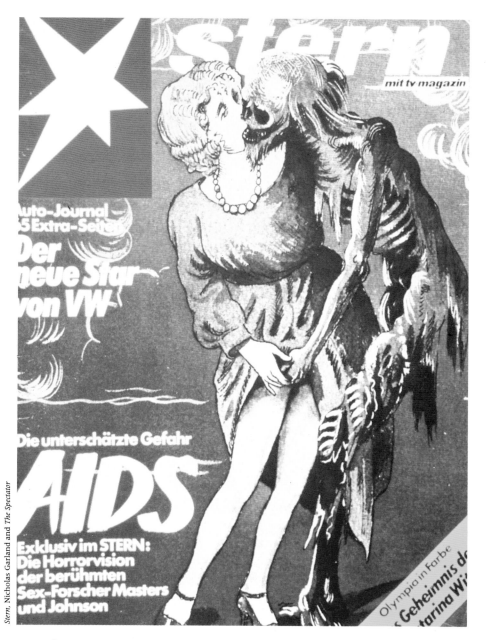

Plate 10

Untitled, Nicholas Garland, 1988.

Drawing from Deutsch's imagery, this 1988 piece featured on the cover of *Stern* magazine, again connects sex and death. Reminding us that AIDS is a sexually transmitted disease, the work also tells us that, as a culture, we have passed this way before.

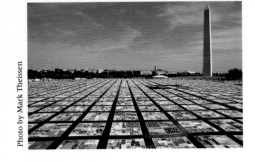

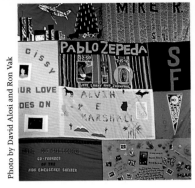

Plate 11 (top left)
AIDS Quilt, various artists, various dates. October, 1992 International Display.

Plate 12 (top right)
AIDS Quilt, various artists, various dates. Close-up of single panel.

The NAMES Project AIDS Memorial Quilt is the world's most visible symbol of the human impact of the AIDS pandemic. The Quilt includes over 26,000 3-foot by 6-foot panels, each commemorating someone who has died of AIDS. Portions of the Quilt are displayed over two hundred times yearly throughout the nation to help increase public awareness of the pandemic. Through its unique ability to touch people's lives and inspire compassion, the Quilt is one of the most effective tools in the fight against HIV and AIDS.

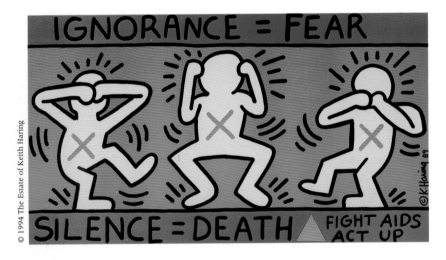

Plate 13
Untitled, Keith Haring, 1989.
Appropriating the well-known image of the three foolish monkeys from the mausoleum in Nikko, Japan, this work admonishes us to hear, see and speak openly and truthfully about the AIDS epidemic. The pink triangle was the symbol for male homosexuals in the Nazi concentration camps and was adopted (and inverted) by the political action group, ACT UP, to emphasize the importance of speaking out—especially during the devastation of the AIDS epidemic.

Notes

1. G. H. Friedland and R. S. Klein, "Transmission of the Human Immunodeficiency Virus," *New England Journal of Medicine*, vol. 317, no. 18 (Oct. 29, 1987): 1125–35.
J. W. Curran, J. M. Mann, P. Piot and T. C. Quinn, "AIDS in Africa: An Epidemiologic Paradigm," *Science*, vol. 234, no. 4779 (November 21, 1986): 955–63.

2. Randy Shilts, "Glory Days," *And The Band Played On* (New York: St. Martins Press, 1987), 11–12. (It is not possible to know with certainty how and when the virus came to America. Randy Shilts gives a reasonable account of this uncertain event and explains the vulnerability of the homosexual community to such an infectious agent.)

3. R. R. Redfield, "Heterosexual Transmission of Human T. Lymphotropic Virus Type III: Syphilis Revisited," *Mount Sinai Journal of Medicine*, vol. 53, no. 8 (Dec. 1986): 592–97.

4. J. J. Roberts, J. R. Robertson and C. A. Skidmore, "The Dynamics of an Illicit Drug Scene," *Scottish Medical Journal*, vol. 33, no. 4 (Aug. 1988): 293.

5. A. B. Bucknall, J. R. Robertson and P. D. Welsby, "Epidemic of AIDS Related Virus (HTLV-III/LAV) Infection Among Intravenous Drug Abusers," *British Medical Journal—Clinical Research*, vol. 292, no. 6519 (Feb. 22, 1986): 527–29.

6. R. P. Brettle, S. Burns and K. Bisset, "Human Immunodeficiency Virus and Drug Misuse: The Edinburgh Experience," *British Medical Journal—Clinical Research*, vol. 295, no. 6595, (Aug. 15, 1987): 421–23.

7. Willard Cates, "The 'Other STDs': Do They Really Matter?" *Journal of the American Medical Association*, vol. 259, no. 24 (June 24, 1988): 3606–08.

8. L. H. Smith and J. B. Wygaarden, *Cecil Textbook of Medicine* (Philadelphia, W. B. Saunders, 1988): 1722.

9. A. S. Benenson, ed., "Control of Communicable Diseases in Man," *American Public Health Association*, 13th ed. (1980), 342.

H. W. Gantt, "A Medical Review of Soviet Russia—IV Change in Type and Incidence of Disease," *British Medical Journal*, vol 2, (July–Dec. 1926): 303–07.

10. Update: "Heterosexual Transmission of Acquired Immunodeficiency Syndrome and Human Immunodeficiency Virus Infection—United States," *Morbidity and Mortality Weekly Report (MMWR)*. vol 38, no. 24 (June 23, 1989): 429–34.

11. P. D. Markham, R. R. Redfield and S. Z. Salahuddin, "Frequent Transmission of HTLV-III Among Spouses of Patients with AIDS-related Complex and AIDS," *Journal of the American Medical Association*, vol. 253, no. 11 (March 15, 1985): 1571–73.

J. M. Jason, R. C. Holman and D. N. Lawrence, "Sex Practice Correlates of Human Immunodeficiency Virus Transmission and Acquired Immunodeficiency Syndrome Incidence in Heterosexual Partners and Offspring of U. S. Hemophilic Men," *American Journal of Hematology*, vol. 30, no. 2 (Feb. 1989): 68–76.

12. N. C. Khan, R. R. Redfield and D. C. Wright, "Correlation of HIV Isolation Rate and Stage of Infection," and abstract THP. 99, p. 180. Third International Conference on AIDS (June 1–5, 1987, Washington, D.C.).

S. Barker, B. Donovan and B. Tindall, "Characterization of the Acute Clinical Illness Associated with Human Immunodeficiency Virus Infection," *Archives of Internal Medicine*, vol. 148, no. 4 (April 1988): 945–949.

13. J. Albert, P. O. Pherson and S. Schulman, "HIV Isolation and Antigen Detection in Infected Individuals and Their Seronegative Sexual Partners," *AIDS*, vol. 2, no. 2 (April 1988): 107–11.

14. K. K. Holmes and J. Kreiss, "Heterosexual Transmission of Human Immunodeficiency Virus: Overview of a Neglected Aspect of the AIDS Epidemic," *Journal of Acquired Immunodeficiency Syndromes*, vol. 1, no. 6 (1988): 602–10.

15. M. Laga, H. Taelman and P. Van der Stuyft, "Advanced Immunodeficiency as a Risk Factor for Heterosexual Transmission of HIV," *AIDS*, vol. 3, no. 6 (June 1989): 361–66.

T. J. Bush, H. A. Perkins and J. W. Ward, "The Natural History of Transfusion-Associated Infection with Human Immunodeficiency Virus. Factors Influencing the Rate of Progression to Disease," *New England Journal of Medicine*, vol. 321, no. 14 (Oct. 5, 1989): 947–52.

16. N. Clumeck, P. Hermans and H. Taelman, "A Cluster of HIV Infection Among Heterosexual People Without Apparent Risk Factors," *New England Journal of Medicine*, vol. 321, no. 21 (Nov. 32, 1989): 1460–62.

17. M. Laga and P. Piot, "Genital Ulcers, Other Sexually Transmitted Diseases, and the Sexual Transmission of HIV," *British Medical Journal*, vol. 298, no. 6674 (March 11, 1989): 623–24.

18. D. W. Cameron, M. N. Gakinya and J. N. Simonsen, "Human Immunodeficiency Virus Infection Among Men with Sexually Transmitted Diseases. Experience from a Center in Africa," *New England Journal of Medicine*, vol. 319, no. 5 (Aug. 4, 1988): 274–78.

R. C. Brunham, J. Pepin and F. A. Plummer, "The Interaction of HIV Infection and Other Sexually Transmitted Diseases: An Opportunity for Intervention," *AIDS*, vol. 3, no. 1 (Jan. 1989): 3–9.

19. D. Greenspan and J. A. Levy, "HIV in Saliva," *Lancet*, vol. 2, no. 8622 (Nov. 26, 1988): 1248.

20. P. C. Fox, A. Wolff and C. K. Yeh, "Saliva Inhibits HIV-1 Infectivity," *Journal of the American Dental Association*, vol. 116, no. 6 (May 1988): 635–37.

21. Anonymous, "Transmission of HIV by Human Bite," *Lancet*, vol. 2, no. 8557 (Aug. 29, 1987): 522.

22. K. Fogel, L. Jacobsberg and S. Perry, "Orogenital Transmission of Human Immunodeficiency Virus (HIV)," *Annals of Internal Medicine*, vol. 111, no. 11 (Dec. 1, 1989): 951–52.

23. D. J. Goldberg, S. T. Green and D. H. Kennedy, "HIV and Orogenital Transmission," *Lancet*, vol. 2, no. 8624 (Dec. 10, 1988): 1363.

24. M. L. Stuber, "Coordination of Care for Pediatric AIDS: The Development of a Maternal-Child HIV Task Force," *Journal of Developmental and Behavioral Pediatrics*, vol. 10, no. 4 (Aug. 1989): 201–4.

25. S. Blanche, M. L. Moscato and C. Rouzioux, "A Prospective Study of Infants Born to Women Seropositive for Human Immunodeficiency Virus Type 1. HIV Infection in Newborns; French Collaborative Study Group," *New England Journal of Medicine*, vol. 320, no. 25 (June 22, 1989): 1643–48.

26. A. Broliden, V. Moschese and R. Rossi, "Presence of Maternal Antibodies to Human Immunodeficiency Virus 1 Envelope Glycoprotein gp120 Epitopes Correlates with the Uninfected Status of Children Born to Seropositive Mothers," *Proceedings of the National Academy of Sciences of the United States of America*, vol. 86, no. 20 (Oct. 1989): 8055–58.

27. S. M. Fikrig, R. Menez-Bautista and S. Pahwa, "Monozygotic Twins Discordant for the Acquired Immunodeficiency Syndrome," *American Journal of Diseases of Children*, vol. 140, no. 7 (July 1986): 678–79.

28. S. E. Hassig, W. Nsa and R. W. Ryder, "Perinatal Transmission of the Human Immunodeficiency Virus Type 1 to Infants of Seropositive Women in Zaire," *New England Journal of Medicine*, vol. 320, no. 25 (June 22, 1989): 1637–42.

29. M. Alam, D. D. Ho and T. Moudgil, "Quantitation of Human Immunodeficiency Virus Type 1 in the Blood of Infected Persons," *New England Journal of Medicine*, vol. 321, no. 24 (Dec. 14, 1989): 1621–25.

30. D. A. Cooper, J. Gold, R. O. Johnson and J. B. Ziegler, "Postnatal Transmission of AIDS-Associated Retrovirus from Mother to Infant," *Lancet*, vol. 1, no. 8434 (April 20, 1985): 896–98.
    Anonymous, "Postnatal Transmission of HIV Infection," *Lancet*, vol. 1, no. 8583 (Feb. 27, 1988): 482.

Anonymous, "HIV Infection, Breast feeding, and Human Milk Banking," *Lancet*, vol. 2, no. 8608 (Aug. 20, 1988): 452–53.

31. W. M. Danker, R. Hatch, R. D. Pratt and S. A. Spector, "Pediatric Human Immunodeficiency Virus Infection in a Low Seroprevalence Area," *Pediatric Infectious Disease Journal*, vol. 12, no. 4 (1993), 304–10.
S. MaWhinney, M. Pagano and P. Thomas, "Age at AIDS Diagnosis for Children with Perinatally Acquired HIV," *Journal of Acquired Immune Deficiency Syndromes*, vol. 6, no. 10 (1993): 1139–44.

32. T. J. Bush, H. A. Perkins and J. W. Ward, "The Natural History of Transfusion-Associated Infection with Human Immunodeficiency Virus: Factors Influencing the Rate of Progression to Disease," *New England Journal of Medicine*, vol. 321, no. 14 (Oct. 5, 1989): 947–52.

33. "AIDS and Human Immunodeficiency Virus Infection in the United States: 1988 Update," *MWWR*, vol. 38, no. S-4 (May 12, 1989): 1–38.

34. P. D. Cumming, R. W. Dodd, J. B. Schorr and E. L. Wallace, "Exposure of Patients to Human Immunodeficiency Virus Through the Transfusion of Blood Components that Test Anti-body-Negative," *New England Journal of Medicine*, vol. 321, no. 14 (Oct. 5, 1989): 941–46.

35. J. E. Groopman, P. D. Markham and S. Z. Salahuddin, "HTLV-III in Symptom-Free Seronegative Persons," *Lancet*, vol. 2, nos. 8417/8418 (Dec. 22, 1984): 1418–20.
M. Krohn, A. Ranki and S. L. Valle, "Long Latency Precedes Overt Seroconversion in Sexually Transmitted Human-Immudeficiency-Virus Infection," *Lancet*, vol. 2, no. 8559 (Sept.12, 1987): 589–93.
D. T. Imagawa, M. H. Lee and S. M. Wolinsky, "Human Immunodeficiency Virus Type 1 Infection in Homosexual Men Who Remain Seronegative for Prolonged Periods," *New England Journal of Medicine*, vol. 320, no. 22 (June 1, 1989): 1458-62.

36. Allan M. Brandt, "The Syphilis Epidemic and Its Relation to AIDS," *Science*, vol. 239, no. 4838 (Jan. 22, 1988): 375–80.

37. Thomas Parran, *Shadow on the Land* (New York: Reynal and Hitchcock, 1937).

38. Ibid., 91.

39. Ibid.

40. Ibid., 92–111.

41. Ibid., 101.

42. Ibid., 103.

43. A. G. Bird, "HIV Infection: The Swedish Approach," *Journal of the Royal College of Physicians of London*, vol. 22, no. 2 (April 1988): 114–17.

44. J. E. Bennett, R. G. Douglas and G. L. Mandell, eds., *Principles and Practice of Infectious Diseases* (New York: Churchill Livingston, 1990), 1214–17.

45. J. H. Hoofnagle, "Toward Universal Vaccination Against Hepatitis B Virus," *New England Journal of Medicine*, vol. 321, no. 19 (Nov. 9, 1989): 1333–34.

Chapter 5

The Cultural Dissemination
of HIV

NEVER IN THE HISTORY OF HUMAN involvement with lenti viruses has science been able to come up with either an effective
cure or an effective vaccine, and it seems unlikely that current
efforts will be rewarded very soon. But we do have access to
another means to control the spread of HIV—prevention. Before
medical technology developed to its current level, epidemics
simply wore themselves out because of changes in society. If we
can deliberately choreograph these changes, we can force an
early end to the HIV epidemic. Unfortunately, a number of cultural inhibitions stand in the way. These inhibitions are rooted in
the fact that, in America, AIDS first showed up in two "socially
unacceptable" populations — homosexual men and drug addicts.

In the 1970s, the new human lenti virus, HIV, was introduced into the gay male culture of America. Male homosexuals in North America had, for decades, suffered discrimination in jobs and housing. Gay bars were almost routinely raided by police, and gay "bashing"—unprovoked violence against homosexuals—frequently occurred. Psychiatrists and psychologists frequently diagnosed homosexuals as mentally ill, solely on the basis of their sexual orientation. Then, in the late 1960s and early '70s, the gay community began to "come out of the closet." Gay men and lesbians began to exert their political power and claim their civil rights. Physicians, lawyers and businesspeople stopped hiding their homosexual orientation. There were marches and parades, and an era of celebration began.

As a result of this new freedom, the bathhouse culture flourished, and anonymous sex became increasingly common within the gay male community. Many individuals explored the limits of sexuality. Condoms, the most effective barrier against the transmission of venereal disease, were rarely used. Syphilis rates rose, as did those for gonorrhea. Intestinal parasites and hepatitis became increasingly common. A group of infectious diseases, primarily but not exclusively spread by anal and oral sex, circulated in the gay male communities of North America.

Eventually physicians with large gay practices began to be concerned about the unhealthy lifestyles and the burden of disease in the gay male community.[1] Resistance to infectious diseases was low. A trial for the new hepatitis B vaccine was deliberately carried out on male homosexuals because they were known to have a very high risk of infection.[2] In the absence of any specific, identifiable new disease threat, the warnings of a few physicians had no effect on the unhealthy aspects of the new gay male lifestyle.

Into this resistance-compromised community came a new sexually transmitted virus, HIV.[3] The invasion was initially not recognized because HIV would cause overt illness only after many years of infection.[4] By the time the causative agent was identified in 1983, many members of the gay male communities in the large cities in the United States were already infected.[5]

We know now that HIV is not normally capable of rapid epidemic spread. It evolved with low infectivity and long host survival in order to live in small, isolated groups. The special conditions existing in the gay community in the 1970s allowed the virus to spread very rapidly in North America. Resistance-compromised gay men with multiple sex partners readily became infected with HIV in the 1970s. Many were already ill with multiple episodes of syphilis or gonorrhea and with chronic infections with the herpes virus, cytomegalovirus, Epstein Barr virus or hepatitis B virus.

The mixing of people in the gay bars and the bathhouses, the mixing of people of diverse economic and social backgrounds and the mixing of well-traveled people with the local crowd spread HIV to every gay male community in every major city of North America.

On June 5, 1981, the Centers for Disease Control of the United States Public Health Service published an article entitled "Pneumocystis Pneumonia—Los Angeles" in its weekly review of disease in the United States.[6] The article heralded the beginning of what is now called the HIV epidemic. There was no hint in the article that a great epidemic was in the offing; there was no special sense of urgency. Rather, a peculiar and unexpected medical condition, an unusual pneumonia, was described in five young homosexual males living in Los Angeles. This was a medical curiosity. The report was published to alert physicians to watch for this condition.

Pneumocystis pneumonia had first been described in malnourished children in refugee camps in Europe after World War II. [7] In the United States, it was a rare condition and occurred almost exclusively in patients with severe medical problems.[8] It was seen most frequently in leukemia patients and in patients with immune systems that had been deliberately suppressed because the patients were undergoing organ transplants.

The usual treatment for pneumocystis pneumonia was a drug called Pentamidine. Because of its infrequent use, it was not an economically viable drug, and the Centers for Disease Control of the U.S. Public Health Service, the CDC, was the only source of the drug in the United States.[9] When Pentamidine was requested to treat young homosexual males without cancer and without organ transplants, the CDC was alerted to this new disease.

Five cases of anything in a country with 230 million plus citizens is a small problem. It was the very unusual nature of the problem that led to the publication of the pneumocystis article in the *Morbidity and Mortality Weekly Report*, the *MMWR*. The last sentence of the article read, "...the possibility of pneumocystis infection must be carefully considered in a differential diagnosis for previously healthy homosexual males with dyspnea and pneumonia." The "gay connection" had begun.

One month later, on July 4, 1981, the CDC reported an additional ten cases of pneumocystis pneumonia in male homosexuals: four in Los Angeles and six in San Francisco.[10] The article also reported twenty-six cases of a rare cancer, Kaposi's sarcoma, in male homosexuals in California and New York City. Two of the Kaposi's sarcoma patients had pneumocystis pneumonia. The twenty Kaposi's sarcoma cases in New York City had all occurred in the past thirty months. Prior to this new cluster, there had been only three cases of Kaposi's sarcoma in New York City in the past twenty years. Additionally, the new Kaposi's sarcoma was in young men and was rapidly progressive, with death sometimes occurring within two years. The old Kaposi's sarcoma was observed only in old men and was compatible with many years of normal life. The report concluded, "Physicians should be alert for Kaposi's Sarcoma, Pneumocystis Pneumonia, and other opportunistic infections associated with immunosuppression in homosexual men."

It was awkward to speak about a condition that took thirteen words to name—Kaposi's sarcoma, pneumocystis pneumonia, and opportunistic infections in male homosexuals with immune suppression. This was shortened to "Gay Related Immune Deficiency" (GRID), which became the new unofficial medical name.

GRID was a remarkably lethal disease, killing about half of the patients within a year of diagnosis. As awareness of this new and deadly disease moved into the public consciousness, it became known as the "gay plague." Public policy came to be influenced by the perception that it was a "gay disease."

On August 28, 1981, an additional seventy cases of GRID were reported in the *MMWR,* but the cause of the GRID epidemic remained obscure.[11] Cytomegalovirus, CMV, was the first viral candidate proposed as the cause of the disease. CMV was present in most of the GRID patients, but it was also present in most healthy gay men and in many heterosexuals. Drug abuse causing an increased susceptibility to CMV was also postulated, but that idea suffered from the same criticism. Most people using drugs were not ill. Only one class of drugs was widely used by gay men and not by other groups. These were the nitrites, compounds that abruptly reduce blood pressure. They were taken to increase sexual pleasure. But nitrites had been used for many years, and this was a new disease.

Two other unusual conditions in gay men were soon recognized. Persistently enlarged lymph nodes with fever, fatigue, night sweats and weight loss were observed in patients in New York City and Atlanta.[12] And four cases of an extremely rare lymphoma, a cancer of the blood, were reported in San Francisco.[13] These seemed to be related to GRID. By June 11, 1982, the CDC had collected 355 cases of GRID.[14] The death rate remained high, and many surviving patients were desperately ill.

On June 18, 1982, the CDC published an exhaustive study of the sexual contacts of GRID patients in the Greater

Los Angeles area.[15] Of the nineteen GRID patients, seventeen had had sex with another of the GRID patients within the last five years or with a partner of one of the patients. The remaining two had frequented the specific sex/bath houses used by other GRID patients. Perhaps most striking, nine of the patients were sex partners of fifteen patients with GRID living in other American cities. One patient with GRID had been a sexual partner of six other patients with GRID. This striking cluster of sexually related GRID patients suggested an agent transmitted by sexual activity between males.

However, not all the data supported this conclusion. Of the first 355 cases, 12 percent were in male heterosexuals, many of whom used IV drugs. Was IV drug use also a method of transmission? And, how could one explain the 4 percent who were heterosexual women not using drugs? GRID was a peculiar name for their disease, however they had contracted it.

On July 9, 1982, the CDC reported thirty-four cases of GRID in five states in male and female Haitians.[16] Some had been in the United States for only a few months when they became ill. One admitted to IV drug use and none reported homosexuality. The mystery deepened.

The following week, three cases of GRID were reported in patients with hemophilia.[17] They had received many infusions of a human-blood-derived clotting factor. This, along with the reports of IV drug use in some patients, suggested a blood-borne etiologic agent.

On September 24, 1982, the disease was given an official name, AIDS—Acquired Immune Deficiency Syndrome, the name it bears today.[18] Almost six hundred cases had been reported, 60 percent of whom had already died. The offending agent appeared to be infectious. It was transmitted by sex, IV drug use and the infusion of blood products. But, in the minds of the public and in the minds of most public officials, it was still the "gay plague," and despite considerable educational effort, it has continued to carry the stigma of the "gay plague." This has made it difficult to convince the people of North America and Europe that the deadly new disease is a problem for everyone, not just homosexual men.

On December 10, 1982, the first case of AIDS caused by a blood transfusion was described.[19] The following week brought the description of four cases of mother-to-newborn transmission.[20] In retrospect, we know that this completed the list of ways that the virus can be transmitted. All that was lacking was the cause of AIDS.

The offending virus was discovered in 1983, in Paris, at the Pasteur Institute by a group led by Luc Montagnier.[21] It was confirmed shortly thereafter by identification in the United States by Robert Gallo's group at the National Institutes of Health.[22] Confirmation was also given by J. A. Levy's group in California.[23] The virus was called LAV, then HTLV-III, then ARV, and now, by international agreement, HIV.[24]

The CDC continued to collect statistics on AIDS cases in the United States and have now reported more than 362,000. But, the CDC statistics are misleading in that they report cases only of AIDS, the terminal phase of HIV-caused disease, not the number of HIV infections. It is the cases of HIV infection that represent the current epidemic. From the time of first infection with HIV until the illness is manifested as AIDS an average of nine years transpires. Some cases will occur earlier, but very few will occur in less than five years.[25] This means that people diagnosed with AIDS in 1981 probably became infected with HIV between 1971 and 1976. It also means that the persons infected with HIV this year, 1994, will not begin to become ill until 1999, and only half will have AIDS or will have died of AIDS by the year 2003. The CDC statistics on AIDS cases tell us what the epidemic was doing ten years ago. We need to know what the HIV epidemic is doing today.

Early in the epidemic, HIV spread rapidly among gay males. They make up 70 percent of the people with AIDS. [26] Their sexual practices appear to have enhanced the transmission of several infectious diseases, among them HIV. Part of the reason appears to be the difference between the way a vagina accommodates a penis and the way an anus accommodates a penis. The vagina can usually accommodate the penis without difficulty. The covering of the penis, the lining of the vagina and the lubrication mechanisms evolved to withstand the repeated thrusting of the penis. Repeated penile-vaginal intercourse normally does not lead to any mechanical or physiological problems.

Although the anus accommodates the penis, the lining of the anus and the rectum do not withstand the thrusting of the penis without some damage. Any kind of break in a defense system of the body permits infections to occur more readily than they normally would. When the rectal mucosa is damaged by the thrusting of the penis, it more readily allows the entrance of disease microorganisms. Syphilis, gonorrhea, chancroid, hepatitis B, giardia lamblia and amoebic dysentery flourished among gay males with multiple sex partners.[27]

Into a setting where such inherently unhealthy sexual practices were common came HIV by an unknown route in the late 1960s or early 1970s.[28] With the damage to the rectal mucosa from sexual trauma and from numerous infections, HIV readily infected sexually active gay men who had multiple partners. The minimum effective dose of HIV to establish infection is not known, but whatever it is, many members of the gay male community more readily met the requirement and became infected.

AIDS has devastated the gay community in the United States, and large numbers of gay men are thought to be HIV-infected though not yet ill.[29] Nevertheless, control of the HIV epidemic in the gay community can be accomplished, for much has already been done. The consistent use of condoms by every man engaging in rectal intercourse and fellatio will halt the epidemic. Condoms are not 100 percent effective in protecting a specific individual during a specific sexual act.[30] However, they will prevent most infections.[31] We do not have to stop all transmissions of the virus to halt the epidemic, just most of them. If transmission is infrequent and irregular, the epidemic will stop.

A rather simple cultural modification—widespread, consistent condom use—would halt the HIV epidemic even without a curative treatment or an effective vaccine. The technology needed to control the transmission of HIV, the latex condom, was invented in 1844. The widespread use of condoms would dramatically slow the HIV epidemic and would eventually save many tens of millions of lives in the First World.[32] The advertising and distribution of condoms in America has been successfully opposed by several groups on the grounds that their availability would encourage sexual promiscuity. They believe that the removal of the fear of pregnancy and the removal of the fear of venereal disease would cause the population to indulge in unbridled sexual activity. However, there is no evidence to suggest that this has occurred in the Scandinavian countries where condoms are widely and freely available as a matter of national policy. We must puzzle over the absence of a government-sponsored, high-powered educational campaign to make condom use the norm during sex, and the absence of a massive free condom distribution program.

The newly developed female condom is another critical medical breakthrough and will eventually save millions of lives if it is made widely available, and in the developing world, the vaginal sponge treated with nonoxynol-9 or a similar virus-killing chemical holds great promise for epidemic control. Like condoms, the sponge will not be 100 percent effective. But, by reducing transmission by as much as 70 percent, the burden of HIV disease in the population can be minimized. For if, by an imperfect method, we are able to keep the incidence of a disease relatively low, then the risk to any one person will be acceptably low.

The lights, the traffic, the noise, the bustle and the hustle of Times Square in New York City belie the personal tragedies of the sex trade for which it is center stage. Women and teenage boys sell their bodies for money and drugs. Probably in about 1980, a gay man in the infectious stage of HIV disease had sex with an IV heroin user or shot drugs with a shared syringe. Perhaps the addict sold his or her body for the money to buy heroin, and then shared a needle with another addict. Many addicts gather in "shooting galleries" where they share needles, a practice that spreads blood-borne transmissible diseases. Into this population, which already consisted of individuals with low disease resistance because of their lifestyle and low social resistance because of police pressure, came the lenti virus HIV—and it spread like wildfire, infecting addicts' lovers and their children.[33]

These latter groups of infected persons are the end product of a chain of HIV infection that had its origin with the decision in 1914 to make heroin use illegal.[34] If heroin had remained legal, the addicts would probably smoke heroin instead of injecting it. It is the act of injecting the drug, not heroin addiction itself, that transmits HIV.

Crack—cocaine base in a rocklike smokeable form—is further lowering the resistance of the ghetto population to HIV infection.[35] Female prostitutes who are cocaine addicts frequently must turn a sexual trick to obtain a single cocaine rock, the effects of which do not last for more than an hour. She may sell her body again and again to avoid the terrible depression of withdrawal. Strung out on drugs, debilitated by the addict lifestyle, willing to do anything to obtain drugs, rarely using any kind of venereal protection, the female crack addict has a lowered disease resistance that rivals that of the starving multitudes of Africa.

Intravenous drug addicts make up the second largest group of patients with AIDS.[36] They account for more than 20 percent of known cases. In North America and Europe, most IV drug users are heroin addicts. Only a few use morphine, cocaine or other substances. Heroin is a chemical modification of morphine that enters the brain more readily than does the morphine molecule. Once in the brain, heroin is converted back into morphine. Injecting heroin gives a faster, higher concentration of morphine in the brain than does injecting morphine. It is the sudden presence of a large amount of morphine in the brain that gives the desired "rush" or high to the heroin addict.

IV drug use transmits HIV through tiny blood transfusions. The blood of the addict may have only a small load of virus, but the method is so efficient that transmission rates are very high.[37] Dirty needle and syringe use is much more effective in transmitting HIV than is sex, including unprotected anal sex. Upon finding a vein, the IV drug user draws blood up into the syringe to confirm that the needle tip is in a vein. The heroin/blood mixture is then injected. The addict once again draws blood up into the syringe to wash out the last of the heroin, for heroin is expensive, and the addict wants to enjoy all of it. The blood coats the inside of the barrel of the syringe, and some remains even after the contents are forced out by the plunger. The syringe is generally not cleaned. It is frequently used in the same manner by several people in rapid succession. Each new user gets some blood from the coating on the inside of the barrel of the syringe, and leaves some blood. The addict using a dirty needle and syringe gets a small blood transfusion from the last several users of the syringe.

IV heroin use and HIV transmission are intimately linked. IV heroin use by males appears to be the leading cause of new HIV infections in the United States at the present time. Areas of high IV heroin use have the highest adult HIV infection rates in developed nations.[38] These areas do not yet have the highest AIDS case rates because the HIV infections have occurred so recently that most addicts have not yet had time to become ill.

The girlfriends and wives of male IV heroin users are the next fastest-growing group with HIV infection. They are acquiring HIV through penile-vaginal sexual intercourse with HIV-infected male sexual partners. These females are not yet ill in large numbers because they have so recently become infected. They are, in turn, transmitting HIV to some 30 percent of their newborn infants.

HIV is also moving into the population of female prostitutes via the IV heroin route. Heroin is not a very popular drug with females. But of those women who are addicts, many turn to prostituion to support their drug habit and will eventually become infected with HIV through the use of dirty needles, syringes and other drug paraphernalia.

When police conduct a sting operation to catch males, called "Johns," seeking sex from prostitutes, they invariably catch a few ministers, doctors and businessmen. Communities are generally unaware that these men frequent prostitutes. All men who patronize prostitutes are at significant risk of becoming infected with HIV. They, in turn, will eventually transmit HIV to their wives and girlfriends. Thus, HIV is filtered through the IV-drug pipeline into the general population. As a result, we pay a formidable price for our self-imposed blindness about narcotics, their use and their control.

Heroin is injected because of the need to use the body as a filter when the heroin is expensive, of poor quality and of uncertain quantity. Given reliable supplies of inexpensive, good quality heroin, addicts don't inject heroin, they smoke it. Smoking heroin is as effective as injecting it for generating the desired high, and it permits better titration of the dose. But smoking wastes heroin. Up to 85 percent is destroyed by heat or is lost into the ambient air. The addict can afford to smoke heroin only if the heroin is of high purity, inexpensive, and reliably available. Needles and syringes do not drive IV heroin use, heroin does. If we change the way we handle heroin, we will change the way the addict uses it. That, in turn, will change the rate of HIV transmission in the heroin-using population. Society can stop HIV transmission among IV heroin addicts—if it chooses.

The severe restrictions on availability of opiates, especially heroin, in the developed nations, are based on false ideas. It is assumed that the ready availability of heroin would lead to a gradually increasing addiction rate in the population. Eventually, so many people would become addicted that the functioning of the society would be dangerously impaired. These ideas about heroin addiction are simply not true. Exposure to opiates rarely leads to addiction.[39] And this is true even when the initial use is non-medical.[40] In America, before the Harrison Narcotic Act halted the free availability of opiates in 1914, one out of four hundred adults was addicted.[41] Most people did not use opiates at all. Long-term opiate use can even be compatible with a productive life.[42] Such addictions cause fewer problems than does long-term alcohol use.[43] Alcohol and opiates were banned at about the same time in the United States. The prohibition of alcohol was repealed because a large percentage of the population had a craving for alcohol. The prohibition of opiates was not repealed because so few people had a craving for opiates.

To stop IV heroin use, we must legalize heroin (or, to use the term invented by the Dutch, "alcoholize"), making it so readily available that no one who needs it has to go without, and so pure that the body is not required as a filter.

Cocaine use is also contributing to the rapid spread of HIV.[44] Most women who become infected with HIV from involvement in the heroin culture acquire the infection from having sex with their HIV-infected husband or boyfriend and not from their own IV-heroin use. Most women who become infected with HIV from involvement in the cocaine culture are themselves cocaine addicts. They acquire the virus through their sale of sex to support the cocaine addiction.[45] The rapid cycle of drug use and drug need (particularly in the crack cocaine society) causes them to have many more sexual partners each day than does a traditional female prostitute. These women with large numbers of customers have correspondingly high rates of venereal diseases: syphilis, chancroid, gonorrhea and herpes.[46] Infection with these diseases appears to increase the likelihood of HIV transmission to a sexual partner. If we provide the drug legally for twenty cents a dose instead of illegally at twenty dollars a dose, cocaine-driven prostitution will probably disappear.

Extracted and purified cocaine chloride is a white, crystalline powder that is soluble in water. It has a temperature of vaporization of 190 degrees centigrade. If heated to this high temperature to be smoked, the cocaine chloride molecule breaks down and has no effect. If cocaine chloride is dissolved in water, mixed with a strong base and extracted with an organic solvent, it becomes a free base. Now the temperature of vaporization is a remarkably low 98 degrees centigrade. It can easily be smoked. Alternatively, cocaine base can be made by adding baking soda to the cocaine chloride powder and heating the mixture. The resulting substance is called crack, after the sound it makes while cooking. It is also called rock because it resembles irregular, small, white stones.

Cocaine in the base form, crack, is heated until it vaporizes, and the vapor is inhaled. This is called crack "smoking" even though the crack is never actually ignited. "Smoking" gives as sudden a high as using cocaine chloride intravenously and allows better regulation of the dose for the desired effect. The recent explosion of crack "smoking" in North

America and Europe reflects the greatly increased availability, purity and low cost of cocaine rather than any innately more addicting property of the crack form.

What percentage of the population is now addicted to cocaine, and what percentage would become addicted if cocaine were both legal and cheap? [47] There is not a precise answer to either question, as the illegal nature of cocaine use makes it impossibly difficult to effectively study the problem. We do know that when cocaine was legal, cheap and readily available—that is, prior to 1914—it did not cause any significant social problems.

Is the threat to our society greater from HIV or from cocaine and heroin use? Will we lose more members of our society from the continued, unchecked spread of HIV through drug users and then into the general population, or will we lose more members of society from heroin and cocaine addiction due to the increased availability of the drugs if they are legalized? The answer is simple and clear. HIV is the greater danger.[48]

The failed policy of drug interdiction and drug suppression has cost the American public staggering sums of money. Federal, state and local costs of criminal sanctions against drug distribution, possession and use amounts to billions of dollars annually. The cost of these efforts has risen steadily since 1914 and is still rising. The money would do much more for the country if spent on roads, schools or even medical research. The benefits of cheap legal heroin and cocaine include reduced HIV transmission and the elimination of a huge criminal empire. They would appear to outweigh any social problems due to increased availability. In a free society with high levels of international trade and travel, it is just not possible to prevent drug use and distribution. IV heroin use and crack cocaine use are rapidly propelling us toward disastrous rates of HIV infection. We do not have time to study the problem. If we are to control the HIV epidemic in America, we must change our drug policy.

Notes

1. J. Robilotti and N. Sohn, "The Gay Bowel Syndrome: A Review of Colonic and Rectal Conditions in 200 Male Homosexuals," *American Journal of Astroenterology,* vol. 67, no. 5 (May 1977): 478–84.
   S. W. DeRamos, Y. M. Felman, H. B. Shookhoff and D. C. William, "High Rates of Enteric Protozoal Infections in Selected Homosexual Men Attending a Venereal Disease Clinic," *Sexually Transmitted Diseases,* vol. 5, no. 4 (Oct.–Dec. 1978): 155–57.
   S. K. Dritz, "Medical Aspects of Homosexuality," *New England Journal of Medicine,* vol. 302, no. 8 (Feb. 21, 1980): 463–64.

2. E. J. Harley, W. Szmuness and C. E. Stevens, "Hepatitis B Vaccine: Demonstration of Efficacy in a Controlled Clinical Trial in a High-Risk Population in the United States," *New England Journal of Medicine,* vol. 303, no. 15 (Oct. 9, 1980): 833–41.

3. The story of the introduction of HIV into the United States and the response of the homosexual community is told in *And the Band Played On,* Randy Shilts, (New York: St. Martins Press, 1987).

4. P. Bacchetti and A. R. Moss, "Natural History of HIV Infection," *AIDS,* vol. 3, no. 2 (Feb. 1989): 55–61.

5. D. M. Lyman, N. Padian and W. Winkelstein, "Sexual Practices and Risk of Infection by the Human Immunodeficiency Virus," *Journal of the American Medical Association*, vol. 257, no. 3 (Jan. 16, 1987): 321–25.

6. The Centers for Disease Control, an agency of the United States Public Health Service, produces a weekly report about diseases in the United States called the *Morbidity and Mortality Weekly Report*, or *MMWR*. It is designed for quick reporting, and more accurately reflects the pace of discoveries about AIDS than do the better known medical journals. The first article was "Pneumocystis Pneumonia—Los Angeles," *MMWR*, vol. 30, no. 21 (June 5, 1981): 250–52.

7. J. E. Bennett, R. G. Douglas and G. L. Mandell, eds., *Principles and Practice of Infectious Diseases.* 3rd ed. (New York: Churchill Livingstone, 1990), 2103.

8. D. J. Krogstad, D. P. Perl and P. D. Walzer, "Pneumocystis Carinii Pneumonia in the United States. Epidemiologic, Diagnostic, and Clinical Features," *Annals of Internal Medicine*, vol. 80, no. 1 (Jan. 1974): 83–93.

9. "Pentamidine Methanesulfonate to be Distributed by CDC," *MMWR*, vol. 33, no. 17 (May 4, 1984): 225–26.

10. "Kaposi's Sarcoma and Pneumocystis Pneumonia Among Homosexual Men—New York City and California," *MMWR*, vol. 30, no. 25 (July 4, 1981): 305–8.

11. "Follow-Up on Kaposi's Sarcoma and Pneumocystis Pneumonia," *MMWR*, vol. 30, no. 33 (Aug. 28, 1981): 409–10.

12. "Persistent, Generalized Lymphadenopathy Among Homosexual Males," *MMWR*, vol. 31, no. 19 (May 21, 1982): 249–51.

13. "Diffuse, Undifferentiated Non-Hodgkins Lymphoma Among Homosexual Males—United States," *MMWR*, vol. 31, no. 21 (June 4, 1982): 277–79.

14. "Update on Kaposi's Sarcoma and Opportunistic Infections in Previously Healthy Persons—United States," *MMWR*, vol. 31, no. 22 (June 11, 1982): 294 and 300–301.

15. "A Cluster of Kaposi's Sarcoma and Pneumocystis Carinii Pneumonia Among Homosexual Male Residents of Los Angeles and Orange Counties, California," *MMWR*, vol. 31, no. 23 (June 18, 1982): 305–7.

16. "Opportunistic Infections and Kaposi's Sarcoma Among Haitians in the United States," *MMWR*, vol. 31, no. 26 (July 9, 1982): 353–54 and 360–61.

17. "Pneumocystis carinii Pneumonia Among Persons with Hemophilia A," *MMWR*, vol. 31, no. 27 (July 16, 1982): 365–67.

18. "Update on Acquired Immune Deficiency Syndrome (AIDS)—United States," *MMWR*, vol. 31, no. 37 (Sept. 24, 1982): 507–8, 513–14.

19. "Possible Transfusion-Associated Acquired Immune Deficiency Syndrome (AIDS)—California," *MMWR*, vol. 31, no. 48 (Dec. 10, 1982) 652–54.

20. "Unexplained Immunodeficiency and Opportunistic Infections in Infants, New York, New Jersey, California," *MMWR*, vol. 31, no. 49 (Dec. 17, 1982): 665–77.

21. F. Barre-Sinoussi, J. C. Chermann and F. Rey, "Isolation of a T-Lymphotropic Retrovirus from a Patient at Risk for Acquired Immune Deficiency Syndome (AIDS)," *Science*, vol. 220, no. 4599 (May 20, 1983): 868–71.

22. R. C. Gallo, M. Popovic and S. Z. Salahuddin, "Frequent Detection and Isolation of Cytopathic Retroviruses (HTLV-III) from Patients with AIDS and at Risk for AIDS," *Science*, vol. 224, no. 4648 (May 4, 1984): 500–503.

M. Popovic, E. Read and M. G. Sarngadharan, "Detection, Isolation, and Continuous Production of Cytopathic Retroviruses (HTLV-III) from

Patients with AIDS and Pre-AIDS," *Science*, vol. 224, no. 4648 (May 4, 1984): 497–500.

23. A. D. Hoffman, S. M. Kramer and J. A. Levy, "Isolation of Lymphocytopathic Retroviruses from San Francisco Patients with AIDS," *Science*, vol 232, no. 4751 (May 9, 1986): 697.

24. J. Coffin, A. Haase and J. A. Levy, "Human Immunodeficiency Virus" (letter). *Science*, vol. 232, no. 4751 (May 9, 1986): 697.

25. P. Bacchetti and A. R. Moss, "Natural History of HIV Infection," *AIDS*, vol. 3, no. 2 (Feb. 1989): 55–61.

26. "Update: Acquired Immunodeficiency Syndrome—United States, 1981–1988," *MMWR*, vol. 38, no. 14 (April 14, 1989): 229–36.

27. W. R. Owen, "Sexually Transmitted Diseases and Traumatic Problems in Homosexual Men," *Annals of Internal Medicine*, vol. 92, no. 6 (June 1980): 805–8.

   W. F. Goldman, Jr., J. S. Marr and R. M. Pomerantz, "Amoebiasis in New York City 1958–1978: Identification of the Male Homosexual High Risk Population," *Bulletin of the New York Academy of Medicine*, vol. 56, no. 2 (March 1980): 232–44.

   A. W. Chow, L. S. Fisher and E. J. Klein, "Anorectal Gonococcal Infection," *Annals of Internal Medicine*, vol. 86, no. 3 (March 1977): 340–46.

28. The earliest case of AIDS in the United States appears to be from St. Louis in 1968, in a 15-year-old black male. There is no known connection between him and Central Africa. It is certainly possible that he had sexual contact with persons from New York City or the West Coast although nothing is known of his sexual contacts. R. F. Garry, A. A. Gottlieb and M. H. Witte, "Documentation of an AIDS Virus Infection in the United States in 1968," *Journal of the American Medical Association*, vol. 260, no. 14 (Oct. 14, 1988): 2085–87.

29. A group of 307 male homosexuals in San Francisco being followed as participants in a hepatitis study went from an HIV-seropositive rate of

0.3 percent in 1978 to 14 percent in 1980 to 47 percent in 1984. N. A. Hessol, P. M. O'Malley and G. W. Rutherford, "Seroconversion to HIV Among Homosexual and Bisexual Men Who Participated in Hepatitis B Vaccine Trials," 4614, book 2, *4th International Conference on AIDS*, (June 12–16, 1988. Stockholm, Sweden).

In Amsterdam, the cumulative incidence of HIV in two groups of male homosexuals rose from 2.2 percent in 1980 to 39 percent in 1987. R. A. Coutinho, E. M. de Vroome, J. Goudsmit and G. J. van Griensven, "Changes in Sexual Behavior and the Fall in Incidence of HIV Infection Among Homosexual Men," *British Medical Journal*, vol. 298, no. 6668 (Jan. 28, 1989): 218–21.

30. "Can You Rely on Condoms?" *Consumer Reports* (March 1989): 135–41. "Condoms for Prevention of Sexually Transmitted Diseases," *MMWR*, vol. 37, no. 9 (March 11, 1988): 133–37.

31. B. Donovan, J. Gerofi, J. Richters, and L. Watson, "Low Condom Breakage Rate in Commercial Sex ," *Lancet*, vol. 2, no. 8626/8627 (Dec. 24–31, 1988): 1487–88.

32. K. M. Wittkowski, "Preventing the Heterosexual Spread of AIDS: What is the Best Advice if Compliance is Taken into Account?" *AIDS*, vol. 3, no. 3 (March 1989): 143–45.

C. F. Clark and M. D. Knox, "Commentary, The Effectiveness of Condoms: An Individual versus a Societal Perspective," *AIDS and Public Policy Journal*, vol. 8, no. 4 (1993): 193–95.

33. D. Hartel, E. E. Schoenbaum and P. A. Selwyn, "Risk Factors for Human Immunodeficiency Virus Infection in Intravenous Drug Users," *New England Journal of Medicine*, vol. 321, no. 13 (Sept. 28, 1989): 874–79.

D. C. Des Jarlais, S. R. Friedman and D. M. Novick, "HIV-1 Infection Among Intravenous Drug Users in Manhattan, New York City, from 1977 through 1987," *Journal of the American Medical Association*, vol. 261, no. 7 (Feb. 17, 1989): 1008–12.

34. The reasons for the passage of the Harrison Narcotic Act of 1914 are explained in "The Harrison Act," *The American Disease, Origins of Narcotic*

Control, expanded edition, David F. Musto (New York: Oxford University Press, 1987), 54–68.

35. M. A. Goldsmith, "Sex Tied to Drugs = STD Spread," *Journal of the American Medical Association*, vol. 260, no. 14 (Oct. 14, 1988): 2009.

36. Des Jarlais, Friedman and Novick, "HIV-1 Infection Among Intravenous Drug Users in Manhattan," *Journal of the American Medical Association*, 1008–12.

37. T. J. Bush, H. A. Perkins and J. W. Ward, "The Natural History of Transfusion-Associated Infection with Human Immunodeficiency Virus: Factors Influencing the Rate of Progression to Disease," *New England Journal of Medicine*, vol 321, no. 14 (Oct. 5, 1989): 947–52.

38. E. Drucker and S. H. Vermund, "Estimating Population Prevalence of Human Immunodeficiency Virus Infection in Urban Areas with High Rates of Intravenous Drug Use: A Model of the Bronx in 1988," *American Journal of Epidemiology*, vol 130, no. 1 (July 1989): 133–42.
    "Update: Acquired Immunodefinciency Syndrome—United States, 1981–1988," *MMWR*, vol. 38, no. 14 (April 14, 1989): 229–36.

39. R. Melzack, "The Tragedy of Needless Pain," *Scientific American*, vol. 262, no. 2 (Feb. 1990): 27–33.

40. D. H. Davis, J. E. Helzer and L. N. Robins, "Narcotic Use in Southeast Asia and Afterward," *Archives of General Psychiatry*, vol. 32, no. 8 (Aug. 1975): Pages 955–61.

41. In 1900, when heroin was as inexpensive and as available as aspirin is now, only 0.25 percent of the population was addicted. V. Cowart, "Control, Treatment of Drug Abuse Have Challenged Nation and Its Physicians for Much of History," *Journal of the American Medical Association*, vol. 256, no. 18 (Nov. 14, 1986): 2465, 2469.

42. D. F. Musto and M. R. Ramos, "Notes on American Medical History. A Follow-up Study of the New Haven Morphine Maintenance Clinic of

1920," *New England Journal of Medicine*, vol. 304, no. 18 (April 30, 1981): 1071–77.

Edward M. Brecher and the editors of Consumer Reports, *Licit and Illicit Drugs: The Consumers Union Report* (Boston: Little Brown and Co., 1972), 33–41.

43. A. T. McLellan. C. P. O'Brien and G. E. Woody, "Long-Term Consequences of Opiate Dependence," *New England Journal of Medicine*, vol. 304, no. 18 (April 30, 1981): 1098–99.

44. C. Stark, "Cocaine and HIV Seropositivity," *Lancet*, vol. 2, no. 8593 (May 7, 1988): 1052–53.

45. Goldsmith, "Sex Tied to Drugs = STD Spread," *Journal of the American Medical Association*, 2009.

46. M. A. Chiasson, E. Elzak and R. L. Stoneburner, "Risk Factors for HIV-1 Infection in STD Clinic Patients: Evidence for Crack-Related Heterosexual Transmission," abstract T.A.P. 112, p. 117, *5th International Conference on AIDS*, (Montreal, June 4–9, 1989).

47. After World War II, amphetamines were sold in Japan as cigarettes are sold in this country. 550,000 people were thought to be chronic users, or about 1 percent of the population. M. Tamura, "Japan: Stimulant epidemics past and present," *Bulletin on Narcotics*, vol. 41, nos. 1 and 2 (1989) 83–93.

Cocaine has essentially the same properties as amphetamine. An experienced cocaine user cannot distinguish between IV cocaine and IV amphetamine in comparable doses. M. W. Fischman, L. Resnekov and C. R. Schuster, "Cardiovascular and Subjective Effects of Intravenous Cocaine Administration in Humans," *Archives of General Psychiatry*, vol. 33 (August 1976): 983–89.

48. C. F. Clark and M. D. Knox, "Effective Drug Enforcement and HIV Transmission: A Modern Paradox," *AIDS Patient Care*, vol 5, no.4 (1991): 168–81.

Chapter 6

Epidemics:
Approaches, Costs and Controls

As the Crusades unfolded in the twelfth century, Europe was experiencing a rapid growth in population. Labor was in excess, the population was straining the limits of food production and marginal lands were brought under cultivation. The free citizens of the Roman Empire had become serfs. Kings, dukes and bishops ruled by Divine Right over their suffering peoples. Kings and dukes used "surplus" people in interminable wars. The bishops and archbishops expended their excess laborers on churches, building the beautiful Gothic cathedrals of Chartres, Reims, Notre Dame, Cologne, Canterbury and Amiens, to name only a few of the most famous.

With labor in excess, real wages sank. The serfs and peasants lived crowded, filthy, miserable lives.[1] The rulers—kings, bishops, dukes and the pope—enjoyed fabulous wealth and power, but they lived among and with their filthy, miserable subjects, who provided them services: cooking, cleaning, washing, child care and sexual pleasure. Whatever infectious diseases the poor suffered were usually passed on to their masters.

By the fourteenth century, the population of Europe had exceeded the carrying capacity of the land given the available techniques of cultivation.[2] The standard of living for the great bulk of the population was low and was continuing to fall. Misery was everywhere. Under those circumstances, a die-off of a large portion of the population following the introduction of "the Pest" in 1348 improved the lot of those who survived. The Black Death had its benefits. With disease rampant, unemployment disappeared.[3] There was a sudden shortage of labor. Serfs simply walked away from their masters and their hereditary obligations to till the land. They walked away to better-paying jobs—still mostly agricultural, but now on the best and most productive land. Real wages rose. With a shortage of labor to cultivate the land, real estate values fell.[4] The cities, which suffered a particularly high death rate, became population sinks, absorbing a constant influx of people from the countryside.[5] As the hereditary leaders and the wealthy in the cities died, they made room for the brightest and best of the ordinary people to rise to the top.

The general level of prosperity for the entire population rose as the goods of the society were divided among fewer people. No longer stifled by the poverty engendered by a population that had outgrown the technology of food production, productivity rose. This was a time of exciting, vibrant social change. The landed classes lost power, and the merchants in the towns gained at their expense. Serfdom vanished. The nutrition and living conditions of the masses improved. The concept of the nation-state began its rise. The arts also flourished, and national languages emerged. The old power structure of church and monarchy was mortally wounded by the epidemic. This was the time of the flowering of the Renaissance, the great burst of artistic creativity that bloomed in the midst of "the Pest."[6]

The organization of fourteenth century European society, economically, socially and politically, made it uniquely vulnerable to invasion by *Pasteureila pestis*. The fabulous wealth of a few, and the abject poverty, misery and filth of the many, made Europe vulnerable to a disease carried by rats and transmitted by fleas. As European society changed in response to the massive epidemic die-off, conditions improved for the survivors. Nutrition improved. Crowding was reduced. Housing became better. The misery and the filth abated. Over a period of some three hundred years, the living conditions for the great mass of the people improved to such an extent that the society was no longer vulnerable to the ravages of *Pasteureila pestis*. "The Pest" has not troubled Europe since 1720.[7]

No medical discovery stopped "the Pest." No procession of flagellants, no burning of Jews, no blaming of the poor. It was the economic, social and political changes brought on by "the Pest" itself that finally stopped the recurrent visitations of plague. Epidemics are egalitarian. The kings and bishops and dukes and lords were no longer threatened by "the Pest" when the living conditions for their subjects improved substantially. Only when the disease no longer affected the poorest and weakest and dirtiest were the kings and bishops also safe. The epidemic of HIV is the same. No one is really safe so long as *anyone* is ill.

Other epidemics provide similar examples. Cholera ravaged Europe and North America during the nineteenth century.[8] Cholera infection is a terrible and degrading way to die. The patient develops severe intractable diarrhea and eventually succumbs to dehydration and electrolyte imbalance. The cholera bacteria is transmitted through water contaminated by human fecal material. The cholera microorganism reproduces massively in the gastrointestinal tract, producing a toxin that causes the GI tract to put out huge quantities of fluid, which departs from the person's body as massive diarrhea.

Cholera was not controlled or eliminated by a vaccine or an antibiotic or any other medical technique. Medical scientists identified the problem of fecal contaminated water. Engineers solved the problem.[9] Once the cholera germ and its transmission were sorted out, the epidemics were stopped by the political decision to spend the money to bring clean water to everyone. A sanitation program—an expensive national program of plumbing that continues to this day—stopped cholera. We pay our water bills and our sewage bills every month without realizing that those bills are actually a health cost.

Cholera is as deadly now as it was one hundred years ago, and it continues to kill people in parts of the world where clean water is not available.

Smallpox had ravaged human populations since before the time of Christ. It is sobering to realize that an effective vaccine against smallpox was available for 171 years before it was used to eliminate the disease from humans. It was a political decision, not a medical decision, that led to the elimination of smallpox. The leaders of the world finally decided to spend the necessary money to stop smallpox. It was a well-known medical technique—Jenner's cow pox vaccination of 1796—that was the contribution of medical science to the eradication program. The coordinated vaccination program by the World Health Organization to eliminate smallpox began in 1967, and in 1977 the last case of smallpox in the entire world was observed in Somalia in East Africa. It took only ten years to completely eradicate the disease from the earth.[10] Yet the question remains: Why did it take more than one hundred years for the political process to make effective use of a proven, well-known medical technique?

Despite enthusiasm for the wonders of modern medicine, it has been the social-political organization and large-scale provision of clean water, vaccinations, plentiful food and sewer systems that have so dramatically extended the life span of humans. This is true in the First World as well as in the Third World. Strangely, health in America is considered to be a matter of individual concern, as though each person is isolated and unaffected by what happens to a neighbor. In truth, health is a community concern because good health requires a healthy environment, and the people in the community are a part of that environment.

If one person has an infectious disease, everyone's health is threatened by that germ. It is to everyone's advantage that no one be sick. This public health perspective is easiest to understand when dealing with children. There is little resistance to the vaccination of children to prevent diphtheria, whooping cough, polio, measles and mumps. It is recognized that the health of one child is very dependent on the health of the other children.

Hepatitis B is a viral disease that is easily transmitted by blood and blood products, and by bodily fluids, including semen and vaginal fluids. Two hundred thousand people are infected with the virus in the United States each year, and 10,000 are hospitalized. Every year 250 die of the acute virus infection, 800 die from secondary liver cancer, and 4,000 die of associated liver cirrhosis.[11] We have a vaccine that is effective in preventing infection with hepatitis B, but it is considered to be too expensive for general use.[12]

Many dentists, physicians and nurses have not been vaccinated against hepatitis B and are not required to be vaccinated against it. Health professionals can and, sometimes, do acquire the virus from their patients. Infected health professionals can and, sometimes, do transmit the virus to their patients. It defies reason that all health-care professionals are not already vaccinated against hepatitis B. Good public health practice would dictate that everyone be vaccinated against hepatitis B.[13] Everyone's health is endangered by the unwillingness to allocate enough money to have everyone vaccinated.

Protecting the health of the public is a function of government. Massively used and produced, the cost of the hepatitis B vaccine should be modest. Must one wait for 171 years, as with smallpox, before the politicians respond? Medical science has made its contribution to hepatitis B control by developing a vaccine. Now, the political leadership must implement an effective program for its control.

But not all of the struggles with epidemic disease have happy endings, even when political support has been strong. Despite generous government funding for research and long-term worldwide political support, the struggle against malaria has not been successful. Today, malaria affects some 200 million people annually, and kills many of them. Attempts to make an effective vaccine against malaria began in the early years of this century, and generations of scientists have worked on the problem. They are still working on the problem.[14]

Vaccines are not the only way to attack infectious diseases. Interference with the transmission of the microorganism can also halt disease. This approach was tried with malaria. The specific type of mosquito that carried the malaria microorganism was sprayed with an insecticide, generally DDT. This was done worldwide. It was temporarily successful, and malaria rates dropped sharply in the 1950s. Then the mosquitoes developed resistance to DDT, and subsequently, to our second and third generation insecticides. Malaria rates went back up to previous levels. Malaria has also developed resistance to one after another of our anti-malarial chemicals. Our scientific efforts, combined with strong political support for many years, have failed to control malaria. The malaria microorganism has adapted biologically to human cultural innovations as rapidly as they have been introduced.

From this consideration of only a few well-known epidemic infectious diseases, it should be apparent that the attempt to control any new infectious disease involves such a large number of unknown factors that a successful outcome is by no means certain. It is necessary to discover the biological properties of the disease microorganism and its techniques of transmission, and then to develop strategies to control it. Political support must be mobilized to support the application of the strategies for control.

Scientists are, by nature, optimistic. One does not usually hear a scientist saying that a problem is unsolvable. If the problem was thought to be unsolvable, the scientist would probably focus on something else. Likewise, if politicians who provide the funds thought that the problem was unsolvable, they would divert the funds to some other use. Every new discovery about some aspect of the problem is treated as the beginning of a breakthrough that will ultimately solve the problem. Sometimes, the scientists are correct in their optimistic predictions, and sometimes they are not correct.

The optimistic prediction by scientists that smallpox could be eliminated from humans was accurate. Once the politicians were convinced, it took only ten years to accomplish the task. The optimistic predictions by scientists that malaria could be controlled were wrong. Despite enormous expenditures of money over a period of ninety years, malaria is as terrible today as it was in 1900. The scientists who predicted the control of malaria, and who spent their lives to make that prediction a reality, were as honest and smart as the scientists involved with smallpox; their *predictions* were wrong.

In 1971, the optimism of the medical and scientific community about an impending cure for cancer was so great that the United States congress created a National Cancer Plan, a sort of crash effort to find the cause and cure of cancer. Billions of dollars later, we now realize that cancer has many causes, and few new treatments have been developed. A cure for cancer remains elusive. The improvements in survival of cancer patients is almost exclusively due to technical improvements in the detection of cancer. The technical improvements permit earlier detection, which makes traditional treatments more effective. Ironically, the technical improvements in detection are almost exclusively the result of non-cancer-related research.

That there have probably been as many scientific failures as successes should not cause us any alarm. It rather reminds us that we would be unwise to assume a healthy future that was based upon any one scientific prediction. An announcement by a large number of reputable scientists and responsible government officials that a breakthrough is about to be made does not make the breakthrough happen. The repetitive predictions by medical scientists and government officials that an effective HIV vaccine was just around the corner did not make it happen. They were just predictions by optimistic people. Neither the authority of the scientist nor the rank of the official made it more likely to occur.

We remember the successful scientific predictions and forget the unsuccessful ones. There have been so many of these scientific predictions that have come true, and that have had a major impact on our lives, that we have come to believe in and virtually to worship science. We now put much of our faith in science to solve the problems of the world, whereas our ancestors put their faith in God. But even as God did not save the faithful from dying of the Black Death in the fourteenth century, science may not save us from the ravages of the HIV epidemic, despite the optimistic predictions of scientists and politicians.

Even if science provides us with a useful vaccine or an effective treatment, there is no assurance that we will have the political will to apply it effectively. Even when our scientific information is quite clear, it may be difficult to translate that information into social policy because of conflicting religious beliefs or social customs. The reduction of transmission of sexually transmitted diseases with the use of condoms is well known. The moral opposition to the use of condoms, both to prevent pregnancy and to prevent venereal disease, is also well known.

The extent of an epidemic, its severity in a population, is dependent upon the biology of the microorganism and the cultural context in which it occurs. The course of an epidemic can be altered by interfering with the biology of the organism, by modifying our culture, or by some combination of the two.

Modifying the culture can control or prevent disease, but is generally difficult to accomplish. Bubonic plague and leprosy were both eliminated from Europe by the general improvement in living conditions in response to the population die-back from bubonic plague itself. Cholera was eliminated with plumbing. Smallpox was eradicated by a political program of universal vaccination. There are many different approaches that a culture can take to adapt to a new infectious disease. Social programs can be designed to limit the spread of the microorganism or to mitigate the suffering it causes, but costs and outcomes are uncertain. Science can be recruited to develop vaccines or treatments, but political will and social changes are required for successful dissemination of these treatments, provided they work. Or the disease can run its natural course and shape the society through illness and death, even as society works to control the course and shape of the disease.

Notes

1. R. M. Swenson, "Plagues, History, and AIDS," *The American Scholar,* (Spring 1988): 183–200.

2. Robert S. Gottfried, *The Black Death, Natural and Human Disaster in Medieval Europe* (London: Robert Hale, 1983), 16–32.

3. W. L. Langer, "The Black Death," *Scientific American*, vol. 210, no. 2 (Feb. 1964): 114–21.

4. John Hatcher, *Plague, Population and the English Economy 1348–1530* (London: MacMillan, 1977), 47–54.

5. Paul Slack, *The Impact of Plague in Tudor and Stuart England* (London: Routledge and Kegan Paul, 1985), 144–69.

6. William H. McNeill, *Plagues and Peoples* (New York: Penguin Books, 1976), 170–74.

7. Slack, *The Impact of Plagues in Tudor and Stuart England*, 322–29.

8. The social and political factors associated with cholera are explored in *Disease and Civilization, The Cholera in Paris, 1932,* Francois Delaports, Arther Goldhammer, trans. (Cambridge, Massachusetts: MIT Press, 1986), 35–38, 171–74.

9. A. Roberts, "Down the Drain: Cholera in Britain," *Nursing Times,* vol. 80, no. 41 (Oct. 10–16, 1984): 40–43.

10. Donald R. Hopkins, *Princes and Peasants, Smallpox in History* (Chicago: University of Chicago Press, 1983), 300–310.

11. *Principles and Practice of Infectious Diseases,* 3rd ed., J. E. Bennett, R. G. Douglas, and G.L. Mandell, eds. (New York: Churchill Livingston, 1990), 1214–17.

12. E.J. Harley, C.E. Stevens and W. Szmuness, "Demonstration of Efficacy in a Controlled Clinical Trial in a High-Risk Population," *New England Journal of Medicine,* vol. 303, no. 15 (Oct. 19, 1980): 833–41.

13. J. H. Hoofnagel, "Toward Universal Vaccination Against Hepatitis B Virus," *New England Journal of Medicine,* vol. 321, no. 19 (Nov. 9, 1989): 1333–34.

14. L. J. Bruce–Chwatt, "The Challenge of Malaria Vaccine: Trials and Tribulations," *Lancet,* vol. 1, no. 8529 (Feb. 14, 1987), 371–73.

E. Marshall, "Vaccine Trials Disappoint," *Science,* vol. 241, no. 4865 (July 29, 1988): 522.

Chapter 7

The Political/Medical Model:
Historical Means
of Organization and Application

In 1793, THREE LEVELS OF GOVERNMENT made Philadelphia their headquarters. Residing in the city were the mayor and the Philadelphia city council, the governor of the state of Pennsylvania and the state legislature and the president of the United States and the congress. When yellow fever struck in August, all these public servants fled, except for the mayor.[1] Philadelphia was to record more than four thousand deaths before the frosts of November ended the epidemic.[2]

With fifty thousand inhabitants, Philadelphia was the second-largest city in the thirteen states then making up the United States. That year it hosted several thousand French refugees from Hispaniola, an island where yellow fever was endemic. The refugees had been driven from their homes by the Haitian slave revolt. The first cases of yellow fever occurred among refugees and sailors. Then the area near the city docks was affected.[3] Neither the agent causing it nor the method of transmission were known. Medical opinion was divided as to whether the plague was caused by corrupt air or an infectious particle. A pile of rotting coffee in the docks area was cited by some as the source of the epidemic.[4] While some of Philadelphia's physicians debated the correct diagnosis, most merchants and about half the physicians fled the town. In the absence of the city council members, the mayor had no authority to spend money to fight the epidemic. With the physicians bitterly divided over diagnosis and appropriate treatment, he could not obtain consistent medical advice.

Benjamin Rush, a signer of the Declaration of Independence, is the best known of the physicians who stayed through the yellow fever epidemic of 1793. His heroism in staying at his post is cited now as evidence that every physician is ethically bound to treat the victims of epidemic disease.[5] The example of his disregard for his own health in the midst of the yellow fever epidemic suggests that physicians today should also be willing to risk their lives.

In truth, the performance of Benjamin Rush was atrocious. Despite the praise given to Rush for staying in Philadelphia and treating paying fever patients, he cared for only a small fraction of those who were ill. His "treatment" probably killed many who would have survived. Rush "discovered" that the proper treatment for yellow fever was massive bleeding and vigorous purging (induced diarrhea).[6] In a patient with high fever and liver inflammation, it is difficult to imagine a worse treatment than blood loss and severe diarrhea. He tried to convince the other physicians remaining in the city of the efficacy of his treatment, but fortunately, most did not believe his wild claims.[7] Had Rush prevailed with his ideas, the death toll would have been truly staggering.[8]

In Philadelphia in 1793, there was no public health system. Private physicians handled all of the yellow fever patients early in the epidemic, and the care provided was chaotic, erratic and ineffective. Although individual physicians often visited and treated patients in their homes, nursing care was nonexistent unless provided by relatives and friends. Additionally, a large number of logistical and social problems were created by the epidemic, which the medical establishment had neither the resources nor the experience to handle.[9] The desperately ill yellow fever patients had to be housed, fed, clothed, medicated, bathed, transported and, if they died, buried. Their families had to be supported. The dead overflowed the cemeteries, and the bodies of the poor began to accumulate. The sick, the dying and the dead overwhelmed the resources of the city, medically, physically, socially and financially. The physicians had neither the organizational skills nor the resources to cope with the deteriorating situation.[10] Extraordinary circumstances required extraordinary responses, which only the government operating a specialized system could provide.[11]

Seeing a lack of centralized organization, the mayor convened a group of concerned citizens. They took charge of the city and mobilized its resources to fight the epidemic. They expropriated a nearby country estate and converted it into a plague hospital. Two French physicians, refugees from Hispaniola experienced with yellow fever, were hired to provide treatment. The citizen group recruited nurses, attendants, patient carriers, cooks and grave diggers.[12] They established an orphanage for children whose parents died of the fever, distributed food to the needy and tended to the social and logistical problems created by the epidemic.[13]

Infectious disease epidemics require this type of specialized knowledge and thoughtful intervention. Benjamin Rush's behavior contrasts sharply with the methodical approach of the city's plague hospital and other services set up by the concerned citizen government. Individual physicians are not trained or equipped to manage patients in an epidemic. The support and organization needed to stem an epidemic can be mobilized only by governments.

The parallels between the yellow fever epidemic of 1793 and the present situation with the HIV epidemic are striking. Today, medical care is fragmented—widely variable in quality and in availability. Social support is rudimentary. Preventive activities are sporadic and uncoordinated. Even the magnitude of the epidemic has not been determined. Governments have not yet recognized the seriousness of the epidemic and have not yet provided effective leadership. Control of an epidemic requires the resources and leadership of government. In 1793, most government officials fled the yellow fever, and the people suffered unnecessarily until concerned citizens took it upon themselves to form an emergency government. In 1994, government officials are waiting for a scientific breakthrough to solve the AIDS crisis. That breakthrough may never come.

The father of medical ethics, the Greek physician Hippocrates, made no mention in his writings of an obligation on the part of the physician to treat everyone who was sick. Sick people had no particular claim on the services of a physician, but once the sick person became a patient of the physician, then the physician was bound by the set of ethical rules.[14] Hippocrates would neither applaud nor condemn the risk that Rush took in caring for patients during the yellow fever epidemic in 1793. Hippocrates would have condemned Rush's treatment of his patients because the Greek physician believed that a physician should do no harm.

A brief overview of the history of epidemics indicates no ethic existed that required physicians to care for sick people. There was neither law nor tradition that required physicians to risk their own lives to care for anyone. During the war between Sparta and Athens in 430 B.C., a terrible plague struck Athens, killing one third of the population. Those who nursed the sick frequently became ill and died. Thucydides, a historian who lived at the time and survived the epidemic, described the action of those physicians who risked their lives to care for patients as neither virtuous nor heroic.[15] In the epidemics that struck Rome in the second and third centuries after Christ, the physicians fled along with most of the wealthy citizens. Galen, the great physician whose writings dominated medicine for a thousand years, also fled from Rome.[16]

During the epidemics in Rome, Christians cared for the sick and dying.[17] Such caring behavior was an article of faith. Jewish and Christian doctrine indicates that illness is often sent by God to instruct or punish; it also indicates that it is everyone's responsibility to care for the sick, even at personal risk, even if those who are ill are strangers or have different beliefs.[18] This ancient tradition did not have any special provision for physicians; it applied to all believers, physicians or not. Thus, the Jewish or Christian physician had the same obligation as the lay Jew or Christian. They were to care for and to visit the sick. Throughout the subsequent history of Europe, many Jewish and Christian physicians took this obligation literally. They cared for the poor, the sick and the dying during epidemics without regard for their own safety. However, these were individual decisions to provide medical care based on individual religious beliefs.[19] There did not ever develop a general medical ethic requiring physicians to care for all sick patients whether or not an epidemic was raging.

The Black Death of the fourteenth century and the repeated visitations of bubonic plague to Europe over the next three hundred years precipitated the development of public health as an entity distinct from treatment of individuals. Public health required the organization and use of social and financial resources as well as medical resources.[20]

The city-states of northern Italy were subject to frequent visitations of the plague in the fourteenth, fifteenth and sixteenth centuries because they used extensive seaborne and land-based trading networks. These city-states pioneered epidemic disease control.[21] Most theories at that time attributed the plague to a malignant conjunction of the planets.[22] God's wrath upon man for collective sins was also advanced as a cause.[23] Astute observers understood its contagious nature. [24]

The pest house or plague hospital, known for centuries as the "Lazaretto," was first developed in Venice. The Church of Santa Maria di Nazaret operated a hospital on an isolated island in the Lagoon of Venice. In response to the thousands of untreated sick and dying during visitations of the plague, the hospital was enlarged and staffed with physicians, attendants, cooks and priests at government expense.[25] Its isolated location reflected the growing belief in contagious transmission. Upon diagnosis of plague by a physician employed by the city health office, the patient was taken to the hospital. Household members of plague patients were also sent to the hospital, for they were at high risk for developing plague and were potential carriers. Ships with plague on board, or those that came from a region where plague was present, were held at Nazaret until it was certain that the sailors were not ill and would not become ill. The holding period for exposed relatives and at-risk sailors evolved into a forty-day time span. (Quaranta, from which the word quarantine is derived, is Italian for forty.)[26]

Quarantine was expanded from people and ships to most commercial goods, especially cloth and clothing. Although rats and fleas were not identified as the carriers of plague until this century, one is impressed that health authorities in the fifteenth century recognized the trade goods and activities that disseminated plague. That the contagiousness of plague was well-recognized is evident from the frequent banning of religious processions and other congregations of people when plague was abroad in a city.[27] For three hundred years, this generated conflict between the Catholic Church and the health boards. The church believed that plague was God's punishment and that only increased religious observance would cause him to relent. The city health boards were advised by permanently employed physicians.[28] They identified the arrival of plague and took action to control the epidemic, despite objections from the church.[29]

In 1382, the Venetian senate decreed that physicians who had fled the visitation of the plague must return to the city or lose their citizenship.[30] This has sometimes been interpreted to mean that physicians had to return to Venice and care for plague patients or lose their citizenship. However, physicians in private practice in Venice were not allowed to diagnose or to care for plague patients. If the physician became infected, he might unknowingly carry plague all over the city.[31] Only specifically designated and specially paid physicians were allowed to see plague patients or even patients suspected of having plague. These physicians were themselves under various levels of quarantine. Their work was dangerous, and because they ran a high risk of infection with plague, they were forbidden to see any other type of patient. Their movements within the city were sharply restricted during the epidemic. They could not support themselves with patient fees under these circumstances, so they were paid a salary by the city. [32] The physicians who had fled the plague in Venice were required to return so that they would be available to care for ordinary illnesses and injuries.

Towns hired physicians, generally young ones who had not yet established a practice, to serve as the plague doctors. They were generally well paid, frequently provided with special quarters, and sometimes arrangements were made for the support of their families if the doctors died of plague.

The northern Italian model of specialized plague care came to be used throughout Europe. The city-state of Milan pioneered the isolation of the families of plague patients in a program of progressive movement through the Lazaretto based on days since exposure. Geographical barriers to the movement of possibly infected people were set up for whole provinces, and elaborate customs and quarantine regulations for goods, especially textiles, were enforced.[33]

The diagnosis, treatment and care of the victims of the epidemic eventually became a highly specialized, government-financed and controlled operation during these seminal years of public health. The public-health model provided special doctors and special hospitals operating under special legislation. This same general approach continued into the twentieth century because it was the only effective way to deal with an epidemic.

In May 1847, the American Medical Association issued a long and detailed code of ethics. It included this now often-quoted sentence fragment, "and when pestilence prevails, it is their duty to face the danger, and to continue their labors for the alleviation of the suffering even at the jeopardy of their own lives."[34] This is now cited as evidence that every physician has a long-recognized obligation to care for the victims of an epidemic. Specifically, it is cited to suggest that all physicians today have an obligation to treat HIV-infected persons.[35]

Such an interpretation of the past places an obligation on all present physicians to treat HIV patients and derives from an apparent desire to handle the HIV epidemic within the existing medical structure. If every physician provides a little care, then the federal government will not have to create and operate what amounts to a socialized medicine program to care for AIDS patients. Private practice would be supported and preserved, and no tax dollars would have to be spent on gay males and drug abusers or on impoverished and diseased members of minority groups.

The foolishness of every physician providing a little care is evident on a moment's reflection. The disease caused by HIV infection is remarkably complex and complicated, and it requires highly trained practitioners to understand and apply the latest treatments, relying on the most recent research. If every physician provided a little care to HIV-infected patients, huge numbers of patients would receive inadequate medical care. Private practice did not work during the Black Death in Venice in the fourteenth and fifteenth centuries, nor did it work during the yellow fever epidemic in Philadelphia in 1793. It will not work for the HIV epidemic in North America in the 1990s.

Epidemics such as AIDS require government leadership, government organization and government resources if the response is to be effective. Individual physicians may perform admirably or even heroically during an epidemic, but physicians do not command the resources nor do they have the organizational apparatus to handle the immense complex problems of an epidemic.

A reading of the 1847 code of ethics in historical and literary context reveals that in time of pestilence, physicians should not flee from where they live and work. They should remain to care for their usual patients with their usual illnesses and injuries, even if that care exposes the physicians to the dangers of the epidemic. It restates the structures imposed by the Venetian senate in 1382.

Ethics do not spring forth instantly in response to a crisis. They cannot be made up on the spot. Ethics are inherited standards of behavior developed over time in response to past needs and problems. The principal ethical issue raised by any epidemic is the question of who will care for the sick and the dying. The present medical system cannot adequately or efficiently care for the ordinary illnesses of our citizens. How can those with AIDS be squeezed into our already overburdened system? There has been a recent effort to promulgate a medical ethic that would require all physicians to care for those infected with HIV.[36] This effort has variously been grounded in morality, virtue and law.[37] The outcome of the ethics debate will profoundly affect the delivery of care to those infected with HIV, and the quality of that medical care. Will all physicians care for a few HIV-infected patients, or will specially trained physicians care for most HIV-infected patients? Will all hospitals provide some care to those with AIDS, or will a limited number of specialized government-funded institutions provide most of the care to the infected?

The answer should be straightforward. *Specially trained physicians, paid by the government, should care for most of those infected with HIV.* The care should be provided at government expense and should occur in institutions specializing in such care. This is the traditional approach to the provision of care during severe epidemics. It became the traditional approach because it was the only practical approach. It is still the only practical approach.

Wealthy persons with AIDS have no difficulty in obtaining medical care in America. Modern authors of books on medical ethics repeatedly discuss the problem of unequal access to medical care and lament the fact that the poor receive inadequate health care. They discuss the inequities of the fee-for-service system of medical care in the United States and propose various alternatives, but nowhere do they mention an ethical obligation of every physician to provide care to everyone who needs it. Economics and politics determine access to medical care, not ethics. As a practical matter, most care provided to the HIV-infected people in America is being given in government hospitals by a small number of young physicians in training. We are repeating (at least in part) the pattern of the past—young physicians are being paid by the government to care for the victims of the epidemic in government-financed hospitals.

The modern pattern of plague care, however, differs from past patterns in two ways. The current plague physicians are not yet receiving extra pay, and the national and state governments have not yet acknowledged their responsibility to pay the costs of the epidemic. Eventually, governments will have to assume the burden of the health-care costs generated by the epidemic. A major epidemic is being squeezed into a poorly managed and inadequate medical system. It will not fit. The magnitude of the health-care needs generated by the HIV epidemic will utterly overwhelm our existing health care resources. As in the past, new physicians must be hired and new facilities created to meet the health-care needs generated by the new epidemic. The present inactivity on the part of government leaders and their failure to learn from the past is increasing the unnecessary suffering of the citizens.

Notes

1. J. H. Powell, *Bring Out Your Dead: The Great Plague of Yellow Fever in Philadelphia in 1793* (Philadelphia: University of Pennsylvania Press, 1949), 55, 107–13 and 173–74.

2. Ibid., 281.

3. Ibid., 15–17.

4. Ibid., 12.

5. R. Patterson, "AIDS: The Duty to Treat, 1988 AMA Position," *Mount Sinai Journal of Medicine*, vol. 56, no. 3 (May 1989): 250–51.

6. Powell, *Bring Out Your Dead*, 77–80.

7. Ibid., 81–84.

8. Ibid., 123.

9. Ibid., 90–113.

10. Ibid., "Crisis."

11. This article provides a historical understanding of the interaction of epidemic disease, physicians and governments. Daniel M. Fox, "The Politics of Physicians' Responsibility in Epidemics: A Note on History," *Hastings Center Report*, vol. 18, no. 2, suppl. (April/May 1988): 5–10.

For a description of the development of public health in America in response to cholera see *The Cholera Years: The United States in 1832, 1849 and 1866*, Charles E. Rosenberg (Chicago: University of Chicago Press, 1962).

12. Powell, *Bring Out Your Dead*, "Bush Hill."

13. Ibid., 173–94.

14. The "Hippocratic Oath" is given on page 67 of *Hippocratic Writings*, G. E. R. Lloyd, J. Chadwick and W. N. Mann, trans. (New York: Penguin Books, 1978).

15. The unabridged Crawley translation of *The Complete Writings of Thucydides: The Peloponnesian War* (New York: Random House, 1951), 109–14.

16. Galen's flight from Rome is recounted on pages 95–96 in *The Hippocratic Tradition*, Wesley D. Smith (Ithaca and London: Cornell University Press, 1979).

17. Albert S. Lyon and R. Joseph Petrucelli, "The Rise of Christianity," *Medicine, An Illustrated History* (New York: Abradale Press, 1978), 264–77.

Arturo Castiglioni, "Christian Dogmatic Medicine," *A History of Medicine*, E. B. Krumbhaar, ed. and trans. (New York: Alfred A. Knopf, 1947), 244–46.

For a discussion of plague as a blessing and the opportunity to serve others, see the "Mortality" and "Works and Almsgiving" of the third century Bishop of Carthage, Saint Cyprian. Pages 195–224 and 225–56 in "Saint

Cyprian Treatises" in Volume 36 of *The Fathers of the Church*, Roy J. Deferrari, ed. and trans. (New York: Fathers of the Church, Inc., 1958).

18. Immanuel Jakobovits, "Attitude to Flight from Plague," *Jewish Medical Ethics, A Comparative and Historical Study of the Jewish Religious Attitude to Medicine and Its Practice* (New York: Bloch Publishing Co., 1959), 10–15.
   Ibid., 106–9.
   Arturo Castiglioni, "Fundamental Concepts of Jewish Medicine," *A History of Medicine* (New York: Alfred A. Knopf, 1947), 64–67.

19. Jakobovits, *Jewish Medical Ethics*, 108–9.

20. Anna M. Campbell, *The Black Death and Men of Learning* (New York: Columbia University Press, 1931), 112–16.

21. Richard J. Palmer, *The Control of Plague in Venice and Northern Italy 1348–1600*, Ph.D. thesis., University of Kent at Canterbury, 1978.

22. The pronouncement of the University of Paris in October 1348 as to the case of the epidemic is found in *The Black Death and Men of Learning*, Anna M. Campbell, 14–17, 39–40.

23. Richard Aldington, trans., "The First Day," *The Decameron by Giovanni Boccaccio* (New York: Garden City Publishing Co., 1930).
   Book of 2 Chronicles, chapter 7, verses 13–14. "When I close the skies and there is no rain, when I command the locust to devour the land, when I send pestilence among my people, then if my people who bear my name humble themslves, and pray and seek my presence and turn from their wicked ways, I myself will hear from heaven and forgive their sins and restore their land."

24. The first quarantine regulation was published at Ragusa in 1377. Campbell, *The Black Death and Men of Learning*, 119.

25. Palmer, *The Control of Plague in Venice and Northern Italy 1348–1600*, 183–89.

26. Ibid., 140–45.

27. Ibid., 65 and 300–301.

28. Ibid., 139.

29. Carlo M. Cipolla, *Public Health and the Medical Profession in the Renaissance* (Cambridge: Cambridge University Press, 1976), 11–66.

30. Palmer, *The Control of Plague in Venice and Northern Italy 1348–1600*, 28–29.

31. Ibid., 241–54.

32. Carlo M. Cipolla, "A Plague Doctor," *The Medieval City*, David Herlihy, Harry A. Miskimin and A. L. Udovitch, eds. (New Haven: Yale University Press, 1977).

33. Palmer, *The Control of Plague in Venice and Northern Italy 1348–1600*, 29–37.

34. "First Code of Medical Ethics (1847)," *Ethics in Medicine, Historical Perspectives and Contemporary Concerns*, Stanley J. Reiser, Arthur J. Dyck and William J. Curran, eds. (Cambridge, Mass.: The MIT Press, 1977), 26–33.

35. "Ethical Issues Involved in the Growing AIDS Crisis by the Council on Ethical and Judicial Affairs," *Journal of the American Medical Association*, vol. 259, no. 9 (March 4, 1988): 1360–61.

36. Ibid.
   E. J. Emanuel, "Do Physicians Have an Obligation to Treat Patients with AIDS?" *New England Journal of Medicine*, vol. 318, no. 25 (June 23, 1988): 1686–90.

37. J. H. Kim and J. R. Perfect, "To Help the Sick: An Historical and Ethical Essay Concerning the Refusal to Care for Patients with AIDS," *American Journal of Medicine*, vol. 84, no. 1 (Jan. 1988): 135–38.
   S. H. Miles and A. Zuger, "Physicians, AIDS, and Occupational Risk; Historic Traditions and Ethical Obligations," *Journal of the American Medical Association*, vol. 258, no. 14 (Oct. 9, 1987): 1924–28.
   D. Geraghty, "AIDS and the Physician's Duty to Treat," *Journal of Legal Medicine*, vol. 10, no. 1 (March 1989): 47–58.

Chapter 8

Politics and Medical Ethics:
The Need for Social Regulation

DESPITE THE PRESCRIPTION GIVEN in the last chapter, recent history indicates that conflict has frequently marred the relationship among those ill with AIDS, government agencies and physicians. The government wants to test drugs to study their efficacy before releasing them, while the dying patient wants the chance of trying the newest, possibly effective drug. The newest drugs, and therefore those offering the greatest hope to those dying of AIDS, are frequently available only if the patient participates in a "medical study." Many of the medical studies are "placebo controlled and blinded." That is, half of the patients are receiving an inactive substance instead of the study drug, and neither the physicians nor the patients know which is being administered. As the end point of these studies is death (practically, if not officially), it requires that the patient have enormous faith in the integrity, honesty and accountability of the government health agencies and the medical profession. History, however, suggests that the AIDS patients should be wary of governments and doctors.

When disaster strikes, it is apparently innately human to require an explanation, a cause. And, if no cause is obvious, humans create one. It is helpful if the chosen cause is something that can be influenced. Better still is a cause that can be directly altered. In 1348, the Jews were chosen as the cause of "the Pest."

Balavignus, a Jewish physician in Thonon, in what is now Switzerland, was accused of poisoning the wells and so causing the horrible deaths newly affecting the town. After being stretched on the rack, he confessed. The deaths, he claimed, were caused by black and red powders which he had thrown into the wells. He also claimed that a poisoned person could infect others with her or his breath or perspiration. Those infected would surely die. Other Jews in the area made similar confessions on the rack. In mid-September 1348, the perfidy of the Jews was a satisfying explanation for the horrible deaths striking one town after another.[1]

The epidemic was the "Black Death" of the fourteenth century. One village would lose half its inhabitants within a few months, while a neighboring village would be spared entirely. Poisoning seemed the only rational explanation. It was believed that only the Jews could carry out such a methodical, well-organized and widespread campaign. After all, the Jews had mocked and beaten Christ and cheered his condemnation. They had refused to heed his message. Now, they were trying to demoralize and destroy his followers. Under torture, Jews were made to confess. A special commission was appointed to enforce a judgment of death against all the Jews. In what is now eastern France, Switzerland and southern Germany, the Jews who had not immediately fled were all burned.

Some of the villages struck by the Black Death in 1348 had no Jews. This was difficult for the authorities to explain unless there was Christian participation in the Jewish plot. Many Christians were accused, arrested and quartered. Others were flayed and then hanged. Some Christians confessed in their dying breaths that they had been paid by the Jews to poison the wells.[2]

In 1348, Jews were made the scapegoat for the epidemic in Europe. In the twentieth century, gay males have been chosen as the cause of the HIV epidemic in America. They are also the scapegoat. While it may be psychologically comforting to blame a disease on a particular minority, it is not helpful in controlling the disease. To attack scapegoats diverts social and political energy into divisive channels, and slows the mobilization of the community for effective action.

When the disease caused by HIV was named the Gay Related Immunodeficiency Disease—GRID—the stage was set for increased social discrimination against homosexuals. They were accused of causing the HIV epidemic and infecting "innocent" people through blood transfusions and blood products. Then, in 1985, a blood test for HIV infection was developed. Because most people infected with HIV were male homosexuals, this objective laboratory test could effectively identify gay males. As a minority that was frequently discriminated against whenever identified, the homosexual community was frightened by the prospect of being involuntarily identified and then persecuted.

Recent historical experience in Europe gave them reason to be alarmed.[3] The Holocaust in Europe that killed six million Jews during World War II had among its origins a program by Nazi physicians to improve the human race through eugenics. If the German people were an identifiable race, they could be improved by applying the principles of eugenics. With the active assistance of the academic community and the medical profession, the party began this program with the sterilization of mentally defective humans and the persecution of male homosexuals.[4] The Nazi party initiated a practical program of racial improvement after coming to power in 1933.[5]

The first stage of the German race improvement program was the sterilization of people who were chronically mentally ill. This included schizophrenics, manic-depressives, chronic alcoholics and the mentally retarded. Special teams of physicians performed the sterilizations. These were presumably done in as painless a fashion as possible. The psychiatrists and neurologists at the mental hospitals chose the subjects for sterilization. There were few protests against the program from physicians and none from the professional organizations of physicians. Between 200 thousand and 350 thousand Germans were sterilized.[6]

While all First World countries discriminated against homosexuals in the 1930s, it was the Germans who pressed the issue to an extreme form. Soon after their rise to power in 1933, the Nazis began a systematic program of arrest, torture and killing of homosexuals.[7] Again, German physicians did not object. No religious groups objected either.

Most of the male homosexuals who were arrested, tortured, and killed by the German state between 1933 and 1944 were blond-haired, blue-eyed Germans. After arrest, the male homosexuals were required to wear a pink triangle as the mark of their sexual identity. In the concentration camps, the pink triangle was even more despised than the yellow star worn by Jewish people.[8]

The rationale for suppressing homosexuals in Germany was straightforward. It was believed that male homosexuals would entice the unwary "normal" males into unnatural acts. Homosexuals thus threatened the German breeding stock and breeding efforts by their entrapment of "normal" males. The exact number of male homosexuals killed by the Nazis is unknown. Many of the records of this holocaust were destroyed or lost, but deaths are thought to number more than twenty thousand.[9]

As the decade of the '30s moved on, the Nazi Party consolidated its power and began to move Germany toward a war economy. Chronic mental patients absorbed significant resources, as did children with birth defects and other abnormalities. They contributed nothing to the state and were potentially detrimental to the genetic well-being of the German race. In the summer of 1939, a program of killing such children was initiated. The children were selected for killing by their physicians.[10]

The parents of these children were told that their child had been selected for experimental treatment. The treatment was described as dangerous, but as holding more hope for improvement than any other course of therapy. The parents were induced to sign a consent form for this new treatment. After examination and observation at the institutes, the children were generally killed by lethal injection. The parents were consoled by the thought that everything possible had been done to help their child, including the latest experimental treatment. The children were killed by physicians or under their supervision. They were killed in hospitals on normal pediatric wards in the midst of children who were being given conventional treatment. An unknown number of children, but in excess of five thousand, were killed.[11]

In a society where perfection of the body and spirit was a national goal, adults with chronic mental illness appeared to be a social burden whose deaths would release resources of food, medicine, heating fuel and housing for the use of the state. In December of 1939, The Foundation for Institutional Care began to gas the mental patients, killing them with carbon monoxide. This was accomplished at six special institutes. Unlike the children who were murdered under the charade of an extensive evaluation, the mentally ill adults were killed immediately upon arrival at the institutes. This program continued until August of 1941, by which time some fifty thousand patients, mostly ethnic Germans, had been slain. Patients were selected for killing by their physicians. The program of purification of the German race began with physicians culling and killing defective Germans, young and old. The mental hospitals were emptied. Few physicians protested; fewer still resigned. Universities and their medical faculties participated.[12]

The experience of the homosexuals, Jews and other persecuted minorities in Nazi Germany was not an aberration in history; similar experiences can occur even in a modern democratic state. In the 1920s, twenty-three states in America passed laws for the involuntary sterilization of mentally ill patients in response to pressures toward social improvement. In 1942, Franklin D. Roosevelt signed Executive Order 9066, which permitted the army to seize anyone thought to be dangerous to the well-being of the United States and to subject them to military penalties.[13] The executive order was implemented by Public Law 503 on March 21, 1942. Neither the order nor the law mentioned race, yet they orchestrated the detention in concentration camps of 112 thousand Japanese-American citizens, 72 thousand of whom were native born. These "dangerous" Japanese-Americans, most of them elderly or children, were permitted to take with them into captivity only what they could carry. Most lost everything they owned through confiscation, theft or forced sale at absurdly low prices. There were no hearings and no appeals. They were herded into concentration camps complete with crowded barracks, barbed-wire fences and armed guards. The United States Supreme Court found these actions to be constitutional.

The "Tuskegee Experiment" provides yet another example. In 1934, the United States Public Health Service set up an experiment to observe the effects of untreated syphilis in blacks.[14] This "experiment" was similar to those performed by physicians in Nazi Germany in that effective treatment was withheld, but different in that patients were not deliberately infected. But while Nazi experiments ended with the end of World War II, the American experiment continued until it was exposed by the press in 1974.

Public Health Service physicians set up a study of the effects of untreated syphilis in three hundred black males in 1934 in Macon County, Alabama.[15] For the next forty years, the United States Public Health Service, with the active cooperation of the Health Department of the State of Alabama and private physicians in Macon County, Alabama, conspired to deprive these men of treatment for their syphilis.[16] They also conspired to obtain their bodies for autopsy when they died.[17] Even after the discovery of penicillin, and after its dramatic curative effects on syphilis were well known, the patients were denied penicillin. The physicians lied to their patients and tried to prevent them from receiving antibiotics for any reason, because if a patient in the experiment obtained antibiotics for another infection, the syphilis would be inadvertently treated.[18] The patients, involuntary experimental subjects, were deliberately allowed to die of the complications of syphilis. Their physicians then obtained their bodies for autopsy studies.

The Tuskegee Experiment was not a secret or clandestine operation. Several generations of United States Public

Health Service physicians and private practitioners participated in the experiment and the deception. Some fifteen papers were published in American medical journals with no attempt to hide what was being done.[19] There is a single letter from a physician questioning the ethics of the "experiment."[20] Eventually, a psychiatric social worker interested the press in this outrageous mistreatment of patients, and the experiment was finally terminated in 1974.[21] No physician was ever punished or reprimanded for participation in this deadly human experimentation.[22]

The systematic killing of defective children, mentally ill patients, mentally defective patients, tubercular and typhus patients, homosexuals, Jehovah's Witnesses, Gypsies, Jews, Russian prisoners of war, Slavic civilians and others by the German people was a horrifying episode in history. But, even more horrifying was the willingness of physicians, intellectuals, lawyers, judges, industrialists and military officers to accept the terrible idea of eugenics, and to carry out its bloody implementation.

Physicians in America have also proven to be morally incapable of resisting dominant social ideas and political pressure, at times to the detriment of their patients. However, physicians are members of society and are subject to the social conditions and prejudices of the society. The many years of education required to become a physician insure knowledge, not wisdom. The physicians of Nazi Germany and America did not protect their patients from discrimination, and they did not object when their patients were killed or denied treatment.

America is now experiencing a deadly epidemic that is concentrated in gay men, IV-drug users and racial minorities—groups already subject to intense discrimination. There are solid historical reasons to be concerned about the fairness of the United States Public Health Service and the American medical profession in treating patients subject to social discrimination. The German and American experiences illustrate that physicians will often do whatever the dominant society expects them to do, even if it violates ethical standards and moral beliefs—even if it directly harms their patients. Physicians have no better moral judgment than do the other members of a society, and no more moral courage.

HIV-infected people cannot rely solely upon physicians or upon the power of medical ethics to ensure good care or even honest care. The solution cannot come from physicians working in unregulated, uncontrolled concert with government. *Instead, HIV-infected people, and those who care about them, must engage the political process and influence social perception to ensure that both the government and physicians provide adequate health care and decent, ethical treatment.*

Notes

1. J. R. C. Hecker, *The Epidemics of the Middle Ages* (London: Trubner and Co., 1859). In the appendix see "Examination of the Jews Accused of Poisoning the Wells," 70–73.

2. Ibid., 74.

3. E. J. Haeberle, "Stigmata of Degeneration: Prisoner Markings in Nazi Concentration Camps," *Journal of Homosexuality,* vol 6. no. 1/2 (Fall/Winter 1980/81): 135–39.

4. Robert Parker, *Racial Hygiene; Medicine under the Nazi* (Cambridge, MA.: Harvard University Press, 1988). Chapters 1 and 2 describe the Eugenics Movement and the adoption of its ideas by the Nazi politicians.

5. Alexander Mitscherlich, *Doctors of Infamy: The Story of the Nazi War Crimes,* Heinz Norden, trans. (New York: Henry Schuman, 1949), 90.

6. Robert J. Lifton, *The Nazi Doctors: Medical Killing and the Psychology of Genocide* (New York: Basic Books), 22.

7. Richard Plant, *The Pink Triangle: The Nazi War Against Homosexuals* (New York: Henry Holt and Co., 1986), 50–52.

8. Eugene Kogon, *The Theory and Practice of Hell, The German Concentration Camps and the System Behind Them,* Heinz Norden, trans. (New York: Berkley Books, 1980), 34.

9. Plant, *The Pink Triangle: The Nazi War Against Homosexuals,* 148–49.

10. Lifton, *The Nazi Doctors: Medical Killing and the Psychology of Genocide,* 48–61.

11. Ibid., 51–62.
Mitscherlich, *Doctors of Infamy,* 114–15.

12. Gerald Reitlinger, *The Final Solution: The Attempt to Exterminate the Jews of Europe 1939–1945* (Northvale, New Jersey: Jason Aronson, Inc., 1987), 128–29.
Gitta Sereny, *Into That Darkness: From Mercy Killing to Mass Murder* (New York: McGraw-Hill Book Co., 1974), 65–69.
Lifton, *The Nazi Doctors: Medical Killing and the Psychology of Genocide,* 62–65, 30–44, 48, 80–95.

Benno Muller Hall, *Murderous Science: Elimination by Scientific Selection of Jews, Gypsies and Others: Germany 1939–1945*, George R. Fraser, trans. (Oxford University Press, 1988), 13, 82–85, 92–93, 99–102. Mitscherlich, *Doctors of Infamy*, 90–103.

13. Morton Grodzin, *Americans Betrayed, Politics and the Japanese Evacuation* (Chicago and London: University of Chicago Press, 1949).

Edward N. Barnhart, Floyd W. Matson and Jacobus tenBroek, *Prejudice, War and the Constitution* (Berkeley and Los Angeles: University of California Press, 1968).

Roger Daniels, *Concentration Camps USA: Japanese Americans and World War II* (New York: Holt, Rinehart and Winston, Inc., 1972).

Anthony L. Lehman, *Birthright of Barbed Wire. The Santa Anita Assembly Center for the Japanese* (Los Angeles: Westernlore Press, 1970), 40, 53 for photographs of guards and barbed wire.

14. James H. Jones, *Bad Blood, the Scandalous Story of the Tuskegee Experiment—When Government Doctors Played God and Science Went Mad* (New York: The Free Press, 1981).

15. The attitudes that led to the "Tuskegee Experiment" can be found in "White Man's Burden," *Shadow on the Land*, Thomas Parran (New York: Reynal and Hitchcock, 1937), 160–81.

16. Jones, *Bad Blood*, 10.

17. Ibid., 142–55.

18. Ibid., 213–14.

19. M. B. Moore, Jr., D. H. Rockwell and A. R. Yobs, "The Tuskegee Study of Untreated Syphilis: The 30th Year of Observation," *Archives of Internal Medicine*, vol 114. (Jul.–Dec. 1964), 792–98.

20. Jones, *Bad Blood*, 204.

21. Ibid., 178–80, 204.

22. Ibid., 206–12.

Chapter 9

Ring Around the Rosy

"Ring around the rosy, pocket full of posies, A-choo A-choo, we all fall down." This rhyme has been sung by children for six hundred years. Despite its association with children's play, it has its origin in a disastrous time in human history. The seemingly innocent children's rhyme and game reveals a story of human horror and tragedy, the greatest mortality of humans in recorded history.[1] The "rosy ring" of the song was the inflamed area around the blackened flea bite wound. "Posies" were the fragrant flowers used to ward off the corrupting air. "A-choo, A-choo" or sneezing referred to symptoms of lung-infected victims, who fell down within hours and died. It recalls the terrible plagues of the fourteenth to seventeenth centuries. One in four people sickened and died in Europe as a result of the plague, and the social, economic, cultural and political changes caused by the epidemic were immense.[2]

Today we face another epidemic, perhaps an even greater one than the Black Death. Our historical experience with epidemics has taught us that infectious disease is not determined by individual behavior, but rather by the behavior of populations and cultures. If we are to stop the AIDS epidemic, we must look beyond the individual and beyond individual behavior, and begin to address the way we organize ourselves as a culture and function as a society.

Just as our culture ultimately determines our vulnerability to infectious disease, the structure and function of a society reflect the political process, and it is the political process that must be engaged in any serious effort to control the HIV epidemic. One organization that explicitly recognizes this truth—and acts on it—has been the homosexual political action group, ACT UP, founded by the New York City author and playwright, Larry Kramer.

Most governments do not appreciate the magnitude of the changes to our social fabric, economic well-being and psychological health that HIV will cause. The gathering storm is difficult for our political leaders to understand because the HIV-infected human takes an average of ten years to become ill, and another two or three years to die.[3] But unless aggressively managed by the political process, this epidemic will spread fear and prejudice over the land and change our lives in unimaginable ways.

It may be that our twentieth century governments are no more capable of meeting the challenge of a major epidemic than were the kings and bishops of the fourteenth century who faced the Black Death. Governments handle best the short-term, external, clearly identified threats such as wars. An epidemic that takes years to develop does not attract the interest and resources of governments. The best predictor of the future behavior of humans and their governments is their past behavior. The record of the political response of governments to previous epidemics is not a cause for optimism.

The solution to the AIDS epidemic is to be found in the political process, not in our scientific establishment or in our medical-care system. Physicians can provide us with an understanding of the illness, and scientists can provide us with medical technology, but only politicians can provide the leadership and mobilize the resources needed to control the epidemic. Medicine and science are impotent without the energy and guidance of the political process. Lenti viruses have not shown themselves to be vulnerable to vaccines. If we wait for a scientific breakthrough to save us from AIDS, we may wait forever.

Even if we had an effective vaccine for AIDS, it would take courageous political leadership to extend comprehensive medical care to everyone (drug addicts, prostitutes and criminals included) who is infected. At this point in time, we have no real effective treatment either, and we have no rational hope of developing one soon. Our antiviral agents against HIV (AZT, DDI and DDC) are so toxic and have so little effect that it is uncertain whether they increase life expectancy at all.

The irony of our American situation, with the HIV epidemic expanding relentlessly, is that we already possess the medical knowledge and scientific technology to *control* the epidemic. We lack only the political leadership and the political courage.

Deadly epidemics have repeatedly ravaged human populations for many thousands of generations.[4] In this century, the building of sewer and water systems, the development of vaccines and the discovery of antibiotics, abruptly brought epidemics to a halt in North America and Europe. The nations of the First World have come to believe that through technology and science they can escape from the epidemics of infectious disease.[5] But the principles of biological evolution predict that new organisms will always evolve to fill new ecological niches. As the natural world and culture are ever changing, this process is never ending. Our increasing human population on this planet of finite size constantly creates new possibilities for infectious disease microorganisms to inhabit humans. Despite our scientific cleverness, we will continue to repetitively experience the invasion of new infectious microorganisms.

People of the First World believe that medical science will save them from the HIV epidemic. Medical science can certainly tell us how we might save ourselves, but the actual "saving" is a political and social process, not a medical one. Science, in the form of medicine, can provide us with the tools to save ourselves, but the culture is the workplace, and the political system provides the energy. Medicine alone is powerless in the face of an epidemic.

Drawing from the lessons of history, we have the knowledge to contain this new epidemic.[6] We already understand the techniques of transmission of HIV and the stages of its life cycle. While we cannot stop it dead because we do not have a curative treatment or an effective vaccine, in the industrialized world we can confine it to a small percentage of the population if we respond appropriately. However, it is not at all clear that we have the social insight and the political will to effectively use our scientific knowledge to control it.

Can we respond to the HIV epidemic now that we have scientific knowledge of the infectious agent? Thus far our response to HIV has been ineffective and unsophisticated. With inspired political leadership, it is possible that we may avoid a great social catastrophe. It is also possible that we are so fundamentally limited by the behavior systems which produce our culture that we may not be able to effectively apply our medical insights.

Condoms for both sexes, if distributed aggressively through an education campaign to make their use the norm during all sexual encounters (unless one wants to conceive a child), would stop sexual transmission of the virus. Some will argue that because condoms are not 100 percent effective, they should not be used. But it is not necessary to stop all transmissions to control an epidemic, just most of them. Vaccinations protect a community even when not 100 percent effective and even when not everyone participates because "herd immunity" protects those who are potentially vulnerable. If most transmissions of a germ are prevented, the disease has trouble maintaining itself in the population. So, imperfect, but widespread condom use can control the HIV epidemic—a solution so obvious and so simple that it is painful to contemplate our failure to utilize it.

The only significant HIV transmission, other than penile-vaginal and penile-anal sex, is transmission by injection of illegal drugs—primarily heroin, but increasingly cocaine. This we also know how to stop. Drugs are injected because they are expensive and adulterated. Provided with a reliable supply of inexpensive, high-quality heroin or cocaine, the addict sniffs or smokes the drug. Sniffing and smoking do not transmit HIV. The "War on Drugs" has not only failed to protect our citizens from drug addiction, but it has also infected tens of thousands of our citizens with HIV through the use of contaminated paraphernalia used to inject expensive, adulterated drugs. There is no medical or scientific solution to this problem. There is only a political solution. We should legalize heroin and cocaine. Fewer citizens would then die of drug effects than now die of AIDS contracted because of IV drug use.

It is not enough to spend billions of dollars on AIDS research and patient care. We cannot buy our way out of this epidemic. Science and medicine cannot save us—only responsible political action can. We have successful examples to follow. The Scandinavian countries are controlling the sexual transmission of HIV through the application of traditional public health programs and an aggressive campaign promoting the use of condoms. They approach AIDS as a social issue rather than a moral issue. They have not eliminated the virus from their countries—that is impossible at this point.

But they have so restricted HIV transmission that AIDS is a modest and stable medical problem rather than a rapidly expanding epidemic.

The Netherlands demonstrated that it was possible to control HIV transmission even in the presence of a large population of already HIV-infected illegal drug injectors. The solution was simple in concept, but difficult in political implementation. The Dutch "alcoholized" heroin. They sought to make heroin as cheap and as available as alcohol. Most Dutch addicts now snort or smoke their drugs rather than injecting them. The Dutch made heroin addiction into a medical issue rather than a moral or law enforcement issue. HIV is not spreading further through the Dutch addict population.

If we continue our "War on Drugs" and our "Moral Crusade" against sex education and the widespread use of condoms, we are condemning ourselves to a rising tide of HIV infection. We have the ability to control the HIV epidemic. The control is based on proven technology and successful examples. Will we have the political wisdom, the political courage and the political leadership to apply our knowledge?

The HIV epidemic is shaping our culture as surely as did the Black Death in the fourteenth century. Plays, poetry, novels, movies, paintings and "the quilt" reflect the influence of the HIV epidemic on our individual lives and on our collective psyche. Its effect on our culture will grow until its influence becomes so pervasive that we will be unaware of what life was like before AIDS.

We have difficulty grasping the enormity of the coming death toll from AIDS because we lack any comparable cultural experience and because the virus spreads so slowly. It is the remarkable lethality of HIV that assures its influence on human history. Essentially everyone infected with HIV will die. A 10 percent HIV-infection rate means a 10 percent death rate. No other epidemic in history has been this lethal. Central Africa is already ravaged, and there are predictions of a decline in population for the entire African continent. The vulnerability of the billions of people in Asia has recently been demonstrated by the startling infection rates discovered in Thailand and India. In South America, the epidemic is sweeping unchecked through Brazil.

In the fourteenth century, the human population in Europe had outgrown the ability of the technology to supply adequate food, and the living standards of the great mass of people fell. Nature corrected itself with an epidemic—the Black Death. Now the human population of the world has outgrown its ability to provide adequate housing, water and sewage treatment for most people. While we have abundant food, the environment is rapidly being degraded. A visit to Mexico City, Cairo or Chicago makes this apparent. The HIV epidemic may correct our excessive population pressure.

We can reasonably expect that HIV, assisted by tuberculosis, will serve as a brake on the world's population over the next several hundred years. With the development of new technologies and new systems of government there will then be a further expansion of the human population. Epidemics have their appropriate place in the natural order. In a broad philosophical sense, AIDS is helping us to regulate our population because we are unable or unwilling to do it ourselves.

HIV was apparently introduced into this country through the male homosexual community. It was identified as a gay disease and a gay problem. The majority of Americans see AIDS as someone else's problem, a pattern repeated throughout the history of epidemics. The English called syphilis the French disease. The French called it the Spanish disease. The Spanish called it the Italian disease, and the Italians attributed it to God. AIDS is called the gay disease, the African disease and the addict disease. AIDS is a disease of humans. We all own it, and we are all responsible for its consequences. It is *our* disease.

In the fourteenth century, most of those who died of the Black Death lived in poverty, but some who died were kings and bishops and wealthy merchants. While infectious disease hits hardest among the poor, it invariably leaks into the middle and upper classes. Outside this country, HIV evolved as a heterosexually transmitted disease. The invasion of the gay community in America by HIV is an example of the leakage of the disease into an unexpected group. The possibility of leakage into the white middle class is present so long as HIV exists in our country. And the more widespread the disease, the greater the vulnerability.

Based on the analogy of pre-penicillin syphilis levels in America, the African-American and Hispanic communities may eventually experience adult HIV infection rates of 20 percent or more, while the white rate may exceed 5 percent. Whatever the racial group or economic class, rates will be highest in the large cities, lower in the towns and lowest in rural areas. Within these broad categories, the distribution will vary widely based on income, sexual experience, place of residence, occupation, travel history, entertainment activities, job requirements and factors not yet identified. But to assume personal safety and the safety of one's children through being white, straight and middle class requires a remarkable ability to deny the reality of AIDS. With the infection rate rapidly growing in our communities, even in our rural areas and small towns, we all have some level of risk, and that risk is growing.

In 1993 there were about forty-five thousand new cases of AIDS in America, with the number expected to grow by 10 percent to 15 percent each year, indefinitely. With expenses exceeding $100,000 per case from diagnosis to death, the cost of AIDS to our health care budget is immense. AIDS has the potential to overwhelm the proposed national health insurance system with escalating costs. By taking large numbers of productive young adults and turning them into health resource consumers and welfare recipients, AIDS aggravates the unfavorable demographics of our aging society.

The terrible epidemics that devastated Rome in the early centuries of Christianity led into that historical period called the "Dark Ages," a time when science and the arts fell silent under the heavy weight of superstition and religious intolerance. The Black Death and the related epidemics that swept back and forth through Europe from the fourteenth to the eighteenth centuries devastated the population and wrung despair from the hearts of the survivors, but it led into that great flourishing of the arts and sciences that we celebrate as the Renaissance. The stress of the AIDS epidemic upon our culture will change us in ways that we cannot yet imagine, perhaps for the worse, hopefully for the better.

The present derives significance from its relationship to the past. As the present is ever new, the need for examination of the past is never ending. We reexamine and reinterpret the past in the light of the present in an attempt to provide meaning and direction for the future. An understanding of human behavior during past epidemics will help us in our developing struggle with HIV.

Historians a thousand years from now will examine and comment upon our behavior and that of our governments, this year, next year and in the coming decades. Let us hope that they will find our efforts to control the HIV epidemic to have been rational, compassionate, reasonable and responsible.

Notes

1. This nursery rhyme was first published in 1881 by Kate Greenaway in *Mother Goose*. James Leasor attributes the rhyme to a description of the plague of *Pastureila pestis* in *The Plague and the Fire*, 130–31 (New York: McGraw-Hill, 1961). *The Oxford Dictionary of Nursery Rhymes*, edited by Iona and Peter Opie, Oxford at the Clarenden Press, 1958, 364–65, disputes the origin as being the plague, but gives no other explanation. *The Annotated Mother Goose*, Rhyme 639, note 116, edited by W. S. Baring-

Gould and C. Baring-Gould, (New York: C. N. Potter Press, 1962), 253, explores the issues, but does not reach any conclusion as to the origin.

2. Leonard Cowie, *The Black Death and Peasant's Revolt* (London: Watland Publishers, 1972), 59–69, 85–102.

3. P. Bacchetti and A. R. Moss, "Natural History of HIV Infection," *AIDS*, vol. 3, no. 2 (Feb. 1989): 55–61.

4. R. J. Doyle and N. C. Lee, "Microbes, Warfare, Religion, and Human Institutions," *Canadian Journal of Microbiology*, vol. 32, no. 3 (March 1986): 193–200.

5. Daniel Thomson, "The Ebb and Flow of Infection," *Journal of the American Medical Association*, vol. 235, no. 3 (Jan. 19, 1978): 269–72.

6. Robert S. Gottfried, *The Black Death; Natural and Human Disaster in Medieval Europe* (London: Robert Hale, 1983), 129–60.

Index